# EATING FOR SUCCESSFUL FA

**Other books by Margaret Gore**

*$10 Family Meals*
*The A–Z of Teenage Health*
*The Arthritis Book*
*Australian Landscapes*
*Coffee Moments*
*The Green Guide*
*The Penis Book*
*Taking Control: A new approach to arthritis*
*Your Baby*
*Your Family's Health*

# EATING FOR SUCCESSFUL FAT LOSS

*Margaret Gore*

ALLEN & UNWIN

First published in 1999 by
Allen & Unwin
9 Atchison Street
St Leonards NSW 1590
Australia
Phone: (61 2) 8425 0100
Fax:    (61 2) 9906 2218
E-mail: frontdesk@allen-unwin.com.au
Web:    http://www.allen-unwin.com.au

National Library of Australia
Cataloguing-in-Publication entry:

Gore, Margaret, 1946– .
  Eating for successful fat loss.

  Includes index.
  ISBN 1 86508 058 6.

  1. Weight loss. 2. Food habits. 3. Low-fat diet—Recipes.
  I. Title.

613.25

Set in 10/15 pt Sabon by DOCUPRO, Sydney
Printed and bound by Griffin Press, Adelaide

10 9 8 7 6 5 4 3 2 1

*To my daughter Lisby for her love, encouragement, honesty and sense of humour—without which this book would never have been written.*

# Contents

Conversion guide    x

Acknowledgments    xii

Introduction    xiii

**Part I    Practical matters**

1 Why you should lose excess body fat    3

*Slimming for health and well-being*    3

*Coronary artery disease*    4

*Hypertension*    5

*Mature onset diabetes*    5

*Osteoarthritis*    6

*Obesity*    6

*Fat cell production*    6

*Are you carrying extra fat or do you just think you are?*    7

2 Why our bodies love fat    10

*The fat quiz*    11

*Our taste for fat*    12

*Barometer of fat in foods*    14

3 Why fat is so hard to shift    16

*Why diets don't work*    17

*The hidden fuel in food*    18

4 Nutrition and weight loss    23

*Vitamin B complex*    25

*Vitamin C*    25

*Vitamin E*    26

*Calcium*    26

*Iron*    27

*Magnesium*    28

*Manganese*    28

*Phosphorus* — 28
*Unsaturated fatty acids (UFAs)* — 28
*The omega fatty acids* — 30
*Fat-watching guide* — 30

5 Exercise and fat loss — 38
*Good fat-burning exercises* — 39

6 Strategies for reducing body fat — 41
*Energy boosting/calming foods* — 42
*Eating properly* — 43
*Eat more slowly* — 43
*Dining out* — 45
*Read food labels carefully* — 47

7 The fat-loss eating plan — 48
*Be a tortoise, not a hare* — 49
*Returning to a natural way of eating* — 50
*The fat-loss eating plan* — 52
*Working out your energy requirements* — 55
*Eating from the five food groups* — 56

8 Low-fat cooking techniques — 59
*Barbecuing* — 59
*Casseroling* — 60
*Grilling* — 60
*Microwaving* — 60
*Roasting/baking* — 61
*Steaming* — 62
*Stir-frying* — 62

**Part II Delicious low-fat recipes**

Introduction — 67

9 Breakfasts — 68

10 Lunch dishes — 77

11  Beef, lamb, pork and veal                          91

12  Poultry                                           114

13  Seafood                                           130

14  Pasta and rice                                    151

15  Vegetable dishes                                  170

16  Salad dressings, sauces, salsas and chutneys      188

17  Snacks                                            201

18  Desserts                                          211

19  Baked treats                                      228

20  Entertaining                                      239

Index                                                 262

# Conversion guide

The measurements I have used in my recipes refer to the standard metric cup and spoon sets approved by the Standards Association of Australia.

## Metric cup and spoon sizes
1/4 teaspoon = 1.25ml
1/2 teaspoon = 2.5ml
1 teaspoon = 5ml
1 tablespoon = 20ml

1/4 cup = 60ml
1/3 cup = 80ml
1/2 cup = 125ml
1 cup = 250ml

## Liquids
1floz = 30ml
2floz = 60ml (1/4 cup)
3floz = 100ml
4floz = 125ml (1/2 cup)
5floz = 150ml
6floz = 200ml (3/4 cup)
8floz = 250ml (1 cup)
10floz = 300ml (1¼ cups)
12floz = 375ml (1½ cups)
14floz = 425ml (1¾ cups)
15floz = 475ml
16floz = 500ml (2 cups)

## Mass
1/2oz = 15g
1oz = 30g
2oz = 60g
30z = 90g
4oz (1/4lb) = 125g
5oz = 155g
6oz = 185g
7oz = 220g
8oz (1/2lb) = 250g
9oz = 280g
10oz = 315g
11oz = 345g
12oz (¾ lb) = 375g
13oz = 410g
14oz = 440g
15oz = 470g
16oz (1lb) = 500g
24oz (1½ lb) = 750g
32oz (2lb) = 1000g (1kg)

## Oven temperatures

|  | Fahrenheit °F | Celsius °C |
|---|---|---|
| Very slow | 250 | 120 |
| Slow | 275–300 | 140–150 |
| Moderately slow | 325 | 160 |
| Moderate | 350 | 180 |
| Moderately hot | 375 | 190 |
| Hot | 400–450 | 200–230 |
| Very hot | 475–500 | 250–260 |

# Acknowledgments

I would like to thank the following for their generous help in the production of this book: Susan Dodd and Yvette Elliott from Sydney Markets Ltd; Jan Lenton and Karen Fyvie from Australian Meat and Livestock Corporation; Yvonne McDonald from the Australian Pork Corporation; the Sydney Fish Markets; Chef Rolf Widmer for allowing me to stand in his kitchen and pester him with questions; the National Heart Foundation; the Commonwealth Department of Health; the Australasian College of Natural Therapies; Dr Sue Carruthers. Also all the chefs, food editors and writers with whom I have worked over the years and from whom I have learned so much.

# Introduction

If you are reading this book, you're obviously interested in losing weight, or more precisely in shedding that extra fat you're carrying. You're probably at the point I was at when I set out to write this book—overweight and tired of the constant war waged against an ever-increasing waistline.

As a journalist working on women's magazines, I've spent the last couple of decades going on every diet ever printed. I was at the *Australian Women's Weekly* when it published the Israeli Army Diet which, of course, we all tried. It didn't work and subsequently the Israeli Army denied all knowledge of it. Then there was the Pasta Diet, the Mineral Water Diet, the Banana and Milk diet. I moved on to *Woman's Day* and tried the Drinking Woman's Diet, and the All You Can Eat (which meant all the apples, broccoli and fish you could eat) diet. I then became editor of *Family Circle* magazine and, I'm ashamed to say, published the Best Ever diet and the Take It Off, Keep It Off Diet.

We now know that diets don't work, and that dieting itself sets you up for gaining more weight in the future. But in those days, regaining weight, with bonus fat, was put down to sloppy eating habits and lack of willpower. Of course, what I had been doing all these years was changing my metabolism, enlarging my fat cells and creating new ones, so that by the time I reached my late forties I had well and truly developed 'middle-aged spread', even though I was eating less and less every year.

Shopping for clothes became a demoralising nightmare—you would think that fitting rooms in department stores would have flattering lighting and trick mirrors to encourage us to buy. Instead, they have 'in your face' mirrors—yes, this is what you really look like without clothes—which reveal every fold of fat and lump of cellulite, from every angle. I can't tell you how often I've fled from those fitting rooms vowing to seriously lose weight and then buy clothes. I was a size 16, verging on 18, and I hated myself for being that size.

I was both lucky and unlucky in the way I carried my weight. You see, I was the classic 'apple' shape, which meant my extra fat accumulated at my waistline instead of on my upper arms, buttocks and thighs. This meant that big shirts and long jackets could disguise my overweight and many people didn't realise my actual size. The downside to this was that I was carrying excess internal fat (the 'apple' shape) which was starting to have very negative effects on my health. I developed hypertension (high blood pressure), and osteoarthritis in weight-bearing joints such as my knees, and was told I would have to be on medication for life. This I was not prepared to accept, and I started to research the two conditions. One stark fact stood out—the biggest contributing factor was overweight. I had to do something about it once and for all. But first I needed to know where I had been going wrong in the past if I were to successfully shed my excess fat—and keep it off permanently.

Through my research I realised that my weight problem began after the birth of my daughter, when I was in my early twenties. Until my pregnancy I had never been over 59kg (130 pounds)—in fact, I had been one of those skinny kids and teenagers who could eat everything and never put on weight. During my pregnancy my weight ballooned. Determined to regain my figure after the birth I went on a strict diet—and I've been dieting ever since.

I do have to confess, though, that both professionally and personally food is my passion. For the past 15 years I've worked as a food writer and editor of cookbooks and food magazines because food and cooking are, for me, among the greatest joys in life. So I not only spend much of my working day reading and testing recipes, but I also find cooking one of the best ways to relax—I gain immense satisfaction in preparing and sharing food with my family and friends. I had comforted myself by the fact that one-time *Woman's Day* food editor Jean Hatfield always advised us, 'Never trust a thin cook!', but at the same time I studied nutrition and struggled valiantly to eat a well-balanced, healthy diet.

When I realised that for my health's sake I would have to lose a substantial amount of weight, I made myself two promises. One, that I was going to find the right way to shed my excess fat and keep it off permanently, and two, do so in such a way as to retain my interest and enjoyment of food.

In the course of my research, I looked at health studies from all over the world. I talked to nutritionists, chefs, medical researchers, dietitians, and slowly I put together this book. When I started, I was medically defined as overweight, now I've lost the weight needed to bring me into the normal weight-for-height range, and I'm eating more than I did before, I have more energy, enjoy shopping for clothes and no longer have to take medication. I have not been alone on this journey—my family and friends have been my guinea pigs—all with equal success. I have had a great deal of help and advice from many health and food organisations, without which I could not have written this book.

So if you're tired of carrying around that excess fat and of being on the diet treadmill, take heart. With some minor changes in your lifestyle—and remember it's your current lifestyle which has given you the shape you have—you will end up losing weight permanently, eating more than you do now, having more energy, sleeping better and getting more enjoyment out of life. Simply follow the strategies outlined in this book and you will attain your goals of a slim figure, greater vitality and self-confidence. The good news is—you have to eat to achieve it.

Good luck and bon appetit!

# Part I

## Practical Matters

# 1  Why you should lose excess body fat

It's an amazing fact that these days the majority of people in the developed world are dissatisfied with their weight and would like to be thinner—even the ones with seemingly perfect bodies! Ask your family, friends and colleagues if they'd like to lose some weight and you'll find few who wouldn't like to be thinner.

The Duchess of Windsor believed that 'you could never be too rich or too thin', an opinion which the Western world seems to have taken as its motto for the rest of the twentieth century. Thinness has become not only fashionable, but somehow entangled with ego, status and self-esteem. It's one of the paradoxes of modern life—those in the affluent West who can afford to eat well admire bodies that wouldn't look out of place in famine-ravaged Third World countries.

It's not just women who are trying to shrink their clothes size. Young men, and older men going through a midlife crisis, are also becoming obsessive about their weight, adopting extreme fitness programs and eating regimes, often to the detriment of their health. And while our ideal beautiful figure wastes away, an ever-increasing number of people in Western nations are becoming overweight and obese—despite the fact that the 'diet business' has boomed in the last few decades to become a giant transnational industry. We live in odd times.

Last century, a well rounded figure was something to be proud of: it signalled affluence and status; it proclaimed that you could afford plenty of food and didn't have to work to maintain your lifestyle. Thinness was equated with poverty and the lower classes. Even 50 years ago people would never have dreamed of commenting if a friend had lost weight, because it was usually taken to be a sign of ill health. Today when people say, 'Oh, you've lost weight,' we say, 'Thank you,' and take it as a compliment! How times have changed.

## Slimming for health and well-being

I'm not going to climb on my soapbox about the fashion, diet and women's magazine industries, but I do want to put the issue of body fat into perspective in terms of overall health.

Firstly, the truth is we need fat in our diet to survive. In fact, we need about 25 per cent of our daily kilojoules to come from fat to:

- provide the essential fatty acids which cannot be synthesised in the body (fatty acids are the building blocks of biological membranes)
- provide the fat soluble vitamins A, D, E and K to keep us healthy
- act as a thermal regulator—providing protection from extreme temperature changes and preserving body heat
- protect vital organs from impact, such as the kidneys, heart and liver
- act as an energy store for lactation and times of illness and famine
- act as a packing material.

Without fat we would simply die. In fact, our body goes to great lengths, and utilises some pretty sneaky tricks, to ensure that it is not deprived of fat. Autopsies on some people who have starved to death have revealed that even they still had some unused fat stores.

However, there is good body fat and bad body fat, and understanding the difference between the two is important for your health and well-being. Good fat is subcutaneous fat which lies beneath the skin and includes fat on our hips, thighs and buttocks. There are very few health risks associated with this type of fat.

The enemy is visceral (internal) fat, which surrounds the organs in the abdomen. It's the fat which gives men their beer bellies and women the apple-shaped appearance that those who have it loathe. One simple, if less than perfect, measure which has been used to indicate a health risk from excess body fat is waist circumference. (It should be noted, however, that this can vary with different populations and racial groups.) How do you rate?

| Sex | Increased risk | Substantially increased risk |
|---|---|---|
| Female | over 80cm (32in) | over 88cm (35in) |
| Men | over 94cm (37in) | over 102cm (40in) |

Apart from giving us a stomach that enters a room before we do, carrying excess visceral fat increases our risk of developing diseases like coronary heart disease, diabetes, high blood pressure, gallstones, stroke and some cancers.

# Coronary artery disease

Coronary artery disease develops when plaques of atheroma—cholesterol-rich fatty deposits—cause narrowing or blockage of the coronary arteries, in turn leading to heart failure. Any gain in weight can lead to a rise in cholesterol. A larger body stresses the heart because it has to work harder to pump blood around a greater overall mass and simply to move it around. Think of how your heart pounds if you have to carry a heavy load of shopping, or when you're lifting weights! When that load is extra body weight, that's how much harder your heart has to work to move you around.

So reducing your overall size by shedding excess body fat, as well as reducing the amount of fat and cholesterol in your bloodstream, will benefit your heart and help ward off heart disease.

## Hypertension (high blood pressure)

It's normal for blood pressure to rise when you experience stress or physical activity, but it soon returns to normal as you rest. If your blood pressure remains constantly high, even when resting, you have developed hypertension. If you are under 65 and your blood pressure is 140/90 or higher each time it is taken, you have hypertension. Blood pressure in people over 65 can be slightly higher and still be normal. Normal blood pressure is generally defined as 120/80. As blood pressure rises, the heart and blood vessels have to work harder to pump the blood through the body.

Over time hypertension can lead to major complications, including heart attack, hardening of the arteries, stroke and heart failure. Left untreated it may eventually cause kidney damage and retinopathy (damage to the retina at the back of the eye). If the condition becomes severe it may also cause confusion and seizures.

Hypertension has many causes, one of which is being overweight, so reducing body fat and overall weight will go a long way to reducing your blood pressure and lessening these health risks.

## Mature onset diabetes

Type II or mature onset diabetes usually develops in people over the age of 40, especially if the person is overweight. It's a serious disease which left untreated can lead to retinopathy, damage to the kidneys and nerve fibres, skin ulcers (which may develop into gangrene), atherosclerosis, hypertension and other cardiovascular disorders.

Unlike insulin-dependent diabetes, which is usually seen in young people, mature onset diabetes results from the reduced sensitivity of insulin target cells. Insulin replacement is usually not necessary but reducing body weight and paying attention to diet are crucial in the treatment and management of this disease. If you have been diagnosed with diabetes you should work with a dietitian to establish an eating and weight loss management plan tailor-made for you.

# Osteoarthritis

Osteoarthritis, commonly referred to as the 'wear and tear' disease, is the result of degeneration of tissue in a joint and the growth of bony spurs (osteophytes) causing stiffness, pain and sometimes swelling.

Being overweight is a contributing factor in osteoarthritis because of the greater stress placed on weight-bearing joints such as the hips, knees and lower back. If you suffer from osteoarthritis, or want to avoid it, then it's really important to keep your weight under control.

Many people who suffer from osteoarthritis have gained great relief or remission from the pain and swelling in their joints simply by slimming down into their normal weight-for-height range.

# Obesity

We often use the terms obesity and overweight as synonyms of one another but medically they are quite distinct. In Australia 9 per cent of men and 11 per cent of women are medically considered obese.

Clinically, if your Body Mass Index (see page 7 for how to calculate your BMI) is between 25–30 you would be described as being overweight; if your BMI was over 30 you would be considered obese. Both overweight and obesity can lead to health problems.

# Fat cell production

There are certain critical times in our lives when our bodies are more likely to gain weight through increased fat cell production and enlargement. If we eat more than we need during these periods, the body produces more fat cells in which to store the excess fat. Once a fat cell is formed it is there for life and you can't get rid of it no matter how much dieting or pummelling of the body you do. These critical times are:

- between 12 and 18 months of age
- between 12 and 16 years of age
- in adulthood if you go on extreme kilojoule-restricting diets
- during pregnancy.

As you grow older your metabolic rate slows and you don't require as many kilojoules for your daily energy needs. If you continue to eat the same way at 40 years of age as you did at 20, then you're going to put on weight, unless you expend a great deal more energy each day than you did at 20!

Gender also plays a significant part in weight problems. Men have a higher resting metabolic rate than women, so they have to eat more to fulfil their daily energy requirements. When women reach menopause their metabolic rate slows further; this can be a time when excess weight appears, even in women who have never had a weight problem in their lives.

Heredity also plays its part—and this is true of both obesity and thinness. Studies have shown that if a mother has a weight problem there is a 75 per cent chance that her children (of both sexes) will be susceptible to gaining excess weight. Similarly, if a mother is thin, there's a 75 per cent chance that her children will be thin.

It's important to remember that this hereditary tendency to put on weight is actually a survival mechanism. If you tend to put on weight easily, you have a more efficient metabolism, which would allow you to survive on less food during famine—it's the people with the most efficient metabolisms who survive in lean times.

Fortunately or unfortunately, depending on how you look at it, in the West this trait is no longer an advantage in normal life. If you ever faced a physical crisis where you were deprived of food, such as being lost in the desert, or at sea, or in times of civil unrest, it would be us 'fatties' who'd survive to tell the tale. However, this isn't much of a defence against the 'thinnies' who say, 'Gosh, you've put on weight,' every time we think we look particularly nice in a new outfit!

Fortunately most of us don't face these extreme calamities, so keeping our bodies at a normal weight is good for us medically, socially and psychologically.

## Are you carrying extra fat or do you just think you are?

If, like me when I started writing this book, you can just grab a handful of fat—almost anywhere on the body—you probably do need to shed some weight. But the best way to tell if you're overweight is to work out your Body Mass Index (BMI), which is your weight in kilograms divided by your height in metres squared ($kg/m^2$). (Quick, grab the calculator!)

For example: if you weigh 75 kilos and are 1.67m tall, then your BMI would be $75 \div 1.67^2 = 26.8$, and you would be medically classified as being overweight. If, however, you were 75 kilos and 1.8m tall, your BMI would be $75 \div 1.8^2 = 23.1$ and you would be classified as normal weight.

| BMI | Definition |
|---|---|
| under 20 | underweight |
| 20.0–24.9 | normal weight |
| 25.0–29.9 | overweight |
| 30.0–39.9 | obese |
| 40 and over | severely obese |

A quicker way to tell if you need to shed extra kilos is by checking your weight against your height in the table below. If you fall within the range shown, you don't need to worry.

### *Weight and height chart (based on a medium frame)*

| Women | | Men | |
|---|---|---|---|
| 143cm | 44–49kg | 155cm | 54–59kg |
| 145cm | 45–50kg | 158cm | 55–60kg |
| 148cm | 44–51kg | 160cm | 56–62kg |
| 150cm | 45–53kg | 163cm | 58–63kg |
| 153cm | 46–54kg | 165cm | 59–65kg |
| 155cm | 48–55kg | 168cm | 61–67kg |
| 158cm | 50–57kg | 170cm | 63–69kg |
| 160cm | 51–59kg | 173cm | 64–71kg |
| 163cm | 53–61kg | 175cm | 66–73kg |
| 165cm | 54–63kg | 178cm | 68–75kg |
| 168cm | 56–65kg | 180cm | 70–77kg |
| 170cm | 58–67kg | 183cm | 72–79kg |
| 173cm | 60–69kg | 185cm | 74–82kg |
| 175cm | 61–70kg | 188cm | 76–84kg |
| 178cm | 63–72kg | 190cm | 78–86kg |
| 180cm | 65–74kg | 193cm | 80–88kg |

1 stone = 6.35 kg; 1 pound = 454g; 1 foot = 30.5cm; 1 inch = 2.5cm

If either your BMI or the weight and height chart indicate that you are within a normal weight range, then be happy—and for goodness sake, DON'T GO ON A DIET! All you'll do is set yourself up for gaining weight later on in your life. If you are unhappy with your body shape, strength training may help to sculpt your curves, but it's important to love what nature has given you—and remember that the rest of us are aspiring to achieve what you have naturally.

If, on the other hand, you've worked out that you do need to shed some weight, then read on.

# 2 Why our bodies love fat

You can blame it all on Mother Nature—you see, she programmed our bodies to like fat. As Darwin explained in his theory of evolution, it was the animals best suited to their environment which survived to reproduce, and so their genes and characteristics were passed on to the next generation—for example, the elephants with the longest trunks survived drought because they could reach the higher branches of the trees; as this genetic characteristic was passed on and on, the elephant's trunk got longer and longer.

It was the same with humans—our history could be described as 'survival of the fattest' as well as the fittest. Those of our ancestors whose bodies had an efficient metabolism (i.e. could burn food as fuel at a lower rate) and stored fat easily were the ones who survived the hard times of famine and war. They were also more likely to reproduce and so pass on these characteristics to the next generation.

The human body also developed another survival technique—whenever it experienced famine, it lowered its metabolism, becoming an even more efficient burner of fuel and, at the same time, triggering a response which would create new and enlarged fat cells as soon as the time of plenty returned. When the famine was over, these fat cells sprang into action, hoarding as much fat as they could, so that when the next famine struck the body had more fuel to live off.

Mother Nature also gave us a taste for fat. Somewhere along the evolutionary path we instinctively realised that after eating fat we didn't feel hungry for quite some time, while hunger returned quickly after a meal of fruit and vegetables. So meat, fish, fowl, nuts and seeds became highly prized foods, especially the fatty parts of animals.

It's only in the last 100 years or so that food has become available to us 'on tap', so to speak. In the West we don't have to work hard to grow, hunt or harvest it. We don't have to last through the famine months of winter. The greatest effort we have to make is to drive to the supermarket and push a shopping trolley around. Our bodies, however, have not had enough evolutionary time to adapt to this situation. So unless we lead physically strenuous lives or maintain a rigorous exercise schedule, most of us consume more fuel each day than we burn up. Over time, that means we gain weight.

## The fat quiz

How much do you really know about the fat you're eating? Try this quiz to find out.

1. Which breakfast choice is lowest in fat?
   (a) a plain croissant
   (b) an English muffin with reduced-fat margarine and jam
   (c) a bowl of toasted muesli

2. Which lunch choice is the lowest in fat?
   (a) ham, cheese and salad in pita bread
   (b) tuna, cottage cheese, celery and nuts on brown bread
   (c) bacon, lettuce, tomato and mayonnaise on white bread

3. Which takeaway food has least fat?
   (a) a deli-style hamburger (no cheese or egg)
   (b) a traditional meat pie
   (c) a large sausage roll

4. Which of the following would reduce the most fat?
   (a) removing all visible fat from 100g rump steak
   (b) choosing 30g reduced-fat cheese instead of full-fat cheese
   (c) removing both skin and fat from 100g cooked chicken

5. Which Chinese dish is lowest in fat?
   (a) beef in black bean sauce
   (b) chicken chow mein
   (c) sweet and sour pork

6. What is the fat content of 100g avocado flesh?
   (a) 32g
   (b) 16g
   (c) 12g

**Answers**

1. b.  (a) 12–17g, (b) 3.5, (c) 4.5–7g depending on brand
2. c.  (a) 21g, (b) 25, (c) 17g
3. c.  (a) 17g, (b) 24, (c) 28g
4. c.  (a) 4g, (b) 3, (c) 8g
5. c.  (a) 17g, (b) 26, (c) 21g
6. b.  (16g)

To understand why we gain extra fat deposits, it's important to understand how our bodies use food. Before it can utilise the nutrients in food, the body has to break it down into its various components. What we put into our mouths is highly complex and it's the job of the gastrointestinal tract to break the food up into simpler units which can be absorbed through the intestinal wall and transported through the bloodstream to provide energy and nutrients to the cells.

As we digest food, it goes through a series of physical and chemical changes. This process begins as soon as we put food into our mouths—and sometimes even before this, when the sight and smell of food triggers the secretion of digestive juices and enzymes. Our mouths water; this fluid secreted from our salivary glands not only moistens the food, making it more easily chewed, but also contains enzymes which begin the process of breaking it down.

Active chemical digestion doesn't really begin until the food reaches the middle part of the stomach, where it is combined with hydrochloric acid, water and more enzymes to break down the carbohydrates, proteins and other nutrients.

The stomach is a highly organised biological structure which sorts out and digests different foods at different rates. It takes between one to four hours for food to pass through the stomach, depending on what type it is; fruit is digested fairly quickly, while complex carbohydrates and proteins take longer and fats the longest of all.

Fat is processed in a different way to other foods. The stomach holds it back so that if it's not required immediately, it can be stored. In a way, the body acts like a miser when it comes to fat. It will expend the fuel in all other foods for our immediate energy needs but hold back the fats so that if it doesn't have to burn them, it can store them away in its fat deposits. That's why eating a high-fat meal at night when your energy expenditure is low is the best way to put on weight!

This means that if you overeat in any day by 1000kJ (238Cals), especially if these are consumed in the evening, your body will save the fat kilojoules and use the other nutrients for its energy needs. It's also harder for the body to convert carbohydrate and protein into fat to be stored—in fact, it has to burn energy to do this—so it's much more efficient just to save the fat and store it directly.

## Our taste for fat

The body also has a couple of sneaky ways of making us eat more fat. Firstly, it has given us a taste for fat—chocolate, butter, cheese, chips, pastries, icecream, there are few among us who can say that we don't like any or all of these foods, or dishes containing them. Even when we eat low-fat foods, they seem more delicious with fat added:

- hot toast—with butter
- prawns—with mayonnaise
- pasta—with a creamy cheese sauce
- waffles—with icecream and chocolate sauce.

And what would corn on the cob, asparagus and new potatoes be without melted butter? We're programmed to like fat and so we eat it at every opportunity.

Secondly, when fatty foods are eaten the brain doesn't recognise the 'full' signal sent to it from the stomach. For example, if you sat down to a salad of greens, capsicum, mushrooms, tomatoes, etc. (no dressing), weighing a total of about 250g (8 ounces), you'd probably start to feel full about halfway through and perhaps push your plate away before finishing it. But how easy is it to wolf down a 250g bar of chocolate or 250g bag of chips and still feel hungry afterwards? In this respect the body is deaf, dumb and blind to our consumption of fat.

Paradoxically, our bodies need some fat in order to metabolise fat and to keep functioning properly. I discuss this in Chapter 4 when I look at how good nutrition is vital for successful fat loss.

The good news is that armed with the knowledge of why we enjoy fat and how it is used and stored in our bodies, we can actually change our eating patterns to fool the 'fat miser' into releasing our fat stores and shrinking our fat cells to achieve an overall leaner body.

---

### Feeling down? Eat a Brazil nut

Yes, that's right. A Brazil nut or two a day will help fight the blues. You see, Brazil nuts are rich in the trace mineral selenium. Studies have shown that people deficient in selenium are more likely to suffer from stress and anxiety than people who get an adequate supply. Most selenium in our diet comes from grains, seafood, cereals and meat, but eating a single Brazil nut a day will ensure you maintain an adequate level of selenium. Other foods rich in selenium are canned light tuna, cooked oysters, sunflower seeds and canned clams.

---

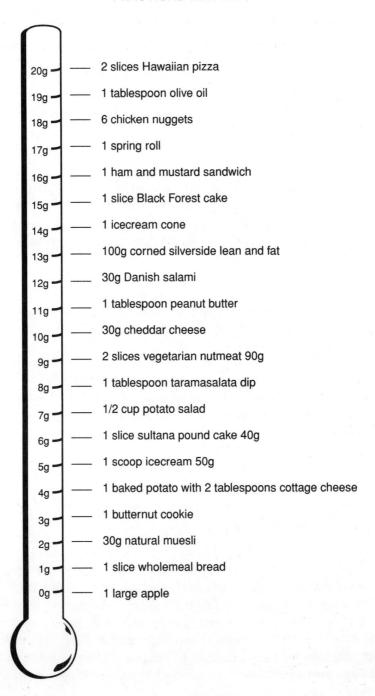

Barometer of fat in foods

## Compare what you can eat for 40–60g fat per day

### WOMEN—40g/5000kJ 1200Cals fat

*Good:*

1 slice rockmelon
1 slice wholemeal toast
1/2 cup baked beans
1 apple
2 slices multigrain bread with mustard, 50g
ham, lettuce, tomato and cucumber
1 peach
1 serve braised beef with Chinese vegetables
100g steamed rice
1 pear

*Bad:*

1 bacon double
cheeseburger

### MEN—60g/9000kJ 2150Cals fat

*Good:*

2 slices wholemeal toast
2 slices ham
1/2 cup baked beans
1/4 cup grated Cheddar cheese
1 banana
1 peach
2 pita pockets
200g lean chicken breast
1/2 avocado
lettuce, tomato, alfalfa sprouts
1 orange
250ml vegetable soup
1 multigrain roll
150g steak
1 large baked potato
1/2 cup mushrooms
1 grilled tomato
1/4 cup corn kernels
1 baked apple stuffed with dates

*Bad:*

1 ham and cheese
croissant and
1 caffe latte

# 3  Why fat is so hard to shift

The reason we all find it hard to lose body fat and keep it off permanently is simply because our bodies don't want us to. As I explained in the previous chapter, the human body will do everything it can to prevent permanent fat loss and goes to great lengths to conserve its fat stores and create new fat cells.

If you go on an excessively low-fat diet, your body will fight back. Its tactics are simple:

- It will give you a craving for fat—have you ever noticed that when you're on a diet you suddenly start obsessing about eating a bag of chips or a chocolate bar, which you would normally never do?
- It will increase your appetite, sending signals to the brain that you are hungry in the hope that you'll consume some fat—that's why when you're dieting you often can't stop thinking about food
- It lowers its metabolism so that it can run on less energy, so any extra food can be stored as fat. It's why dieting progressively lowers people's metabolism, so that when they return to normal eating they regain the weight and usually gain more.

Nature has also made a difference between the way men and women store and use fat—and I'm sorry girls, but we lose out again. A female fat cell is large and prefers to store fat. The male fat cell is smaller and is happier to release its energy stores. This is why women lose less weight more slowly and gain it back faster than men.

There are two types of enzymes responsible for burning or storing fat—lipolytic enzymes which stimulate the body to release fat, and lipogenic enzymes which stimulate it to store fat. Men have many more lipolytic enzymes than women, which makes it easier for males to lose body fat when they take up exercise. Women, on the other hand, produce the female sex hormone oestrogen, which activates and increases the number of lipogenic enzymes. Our large supplies of lipogenic enzymes and fewer lipolytic enzymes make it very hard for us to slim down—our bodies actually resist any loss of body fat.

Nature designed the male of our species to be able to release fat quickly and efficiently, so he has the energy to hunt and fight off invaders. Biologically, he only has to survive three or four winter months of food shortages, and consequently only has to carry enough stored fuel to see him through that relatively short period. Woman, on the other hand, has fat cells designed to store fat quickly and efficiently so she can survive nine months of pregnancy plus at least a year of lactation—this way, she can successfully reproduce despite food shortages. (This original design isn't necessary in the modern Western world, but evolution hasn't caught up with the fact!)

Accepting the fact that permanent fat reduction is going to be a challenge and must be a slow process is half the battle in defeating the bulge.

## Why diets don't work

I've talked about how we inherited our taste for, and ability to store, fat but that's not the whole story. Every time we go on a diet our fat cells go 'Yippee!' because they know they are going to grow and multiply. The feast/famine cycle of our ancestors has become the diet/binge mode of weight cycling today.

It's depressing to think that from the very first slimming diet we tried, we triggered the mechanism that would continually put the weight back on with interest.

Each time we start a diet, our body thinks, 'Wait a minute, I'm not getting the same amount of energy I usually do. Emergency, emergency!' It then triggers the survival mechanism and starts producing lots of lipogenic enzymes to store fat. It drops its metabolic rate so that it doesn't burn as many kilojoules as it did before in order to conserve its fat stores. We may lose weight but it will probably be water and muscle mass because the body wants to burn anything other than its fat stores.

So there you are, you've lost 5 kilos (12 pounds) in weight and are feeling pleased with your achievement. However, unbeknown to you, your body is about to sabotage all your efforts. It's in peak fat-storing mode and ready to pounce. You return to eating what you think is a well-balanced diet and your body springs the trap, stuffing its fat cells, creating more, and making fewer lipolytic (fat-releasing) enzymes—it's making sure it will be better prepared for the next famine/diet. It's a depressing fact that studies have shown that dieting can reduce our lipolytic enzymes by up to 50 per cent.

You despair. You're eating less than you did before and your clothes are getting tighter by the day. It's depressing. It's unfair! Not only have you regained the weight you took so much trouble to lose, but you've put on even more.

You have to accept that energy-restricting diets just don't work—all they do is set you up to become even fatter in the future, because once you have a fat cell, it's yours for life. You may be able to shrink it but you can never get rid of it. Gaining weight by dieting will continue unless you break the cycle.

The good news is you can break the cycle by following the plan outlined in this book. But before I talk about that, let me ask you a question. Do you really know how many grams of fat and kilojoules you consume each day? It's surprising how many of us don't know, so that we can be overeating without really realising it.

## The hidden fuel in food

It's really amazing how many people underestimate their kilojoule intake each day. It's almost as if we have a blind spot for what we eat and simply don't notice the few chips offered by a colleague, the leftovers from children's plates, what we nibble and taste while preparing a meal—but all these kilojoules add up.

I asked many people who said they wanted to lose weight but who also believed that they ate a reasonably good diet, to keep a food diary for just one typical working day. They had to write down absolutely everything they ate, and drank, including chewing gum, coffees, sweets, tastes and nibbles. The results surprised them all. All underestimated the number of kilojoules and grams of fat they were consuming. Here are four typical examples with their kilojoules and fat content added:

*Garry, age 34. Journalist with a sedentary lifestyle.*

|       |                                                    | kJ   | Fat  |
|-------|----------------------------------------------------|------|------|
| 6.00  | tea with milk                                      | 55   | 1    |
| 7.00  | 60g honey toasted muesli                           | 590  | 14   |
|       | 125ml milk                                         | 350  | 5    |
|       | white coffee                                       | 55   | 1    |
| 9.00  | white coffee                                       | 55   | 1    |
| 10.30 | white coffee                                       | 55   | 1    |
|       | 2 chocolate-coated Scotch Finger biscuits          | 970  | 11   |
| 1.00  | 1 wholemeal roll with veal schnitzel and salad     | 2355 | 27.5 |
|       | 250ml flavoured soy milk drink                     | 650  | 8.5  |
|       | 1 large apple                                      | 440  | 0    |
| 4.00  | 1 white coffee                                     | 55   | 1    |
| 6.30  | 1 middy beer                                       | 440  | 0    |

|       |                            | kJ     | Fat |
|-------|----------------------------|--------|-----|
|       | 30g pkt potato crisps      | 630    | 9   |
| 8.15  | 1 serving pork in plum sauce | 2260 | 39  |
|       | 1 cup plain rice           | 775    | 0   |
|       | 1 banana                   | 545    | 0   |
|       | 2 glasses red wine         | 750    | 0   |
| 10.00 | 1 cup white tea            | 55     | 1   |
|       | Total                      | 11 085 | 120 |

Garry's total intake of kilojoules was reasonable but his fat intake was a whopping 120g, double the recommended maximum of 60g for a man. It represented 40 per cent of his total kilojoule intake instead of the 25 per cent recommended allowance. In addition, almost all of the fat would have been saturated fat, very little of it from the mono- and polyunsaturated types.

## Julia, aged 28. Secretary with a generally sedentary lifestyle.

|       |                                                  | kJ     | Fat |
|-------|--------------------------------------------------|--------|-----|
| 7.15  | 250ml orange juice                               | 450    | 1.5 |
|       | 1 skim milk banana smoothie with lecithin and wheat germ | 1160 | 12 |
| 9.00  | 1 large apple                                    | 440    | 0   |
|       | 1 skim milk cappuccino                           | 210    | 0   |
| 10.25 | 4 macadamia nuts                                 | 480    | 12  |
| 12.30 | 1 pita pocket with prawn, apple, celery and mayonnaise | 1630 | 18 |
|       | 200g lite flavoured yoghurt                      | 755    | 0.2 |
|       | 200ml apple juice                                | 390    | 0   |
| 3.20  | 1 honey log health food bar, 45g                 | 1050   | 13  |
|       | 1 herbal tea                                     | 15     | 0   |
| 7.00  | 1 cup Caesar salad                               | 795    | 13  |
|       | 1/2 cup fresh fruit salad                        | 250    | 0   |
|       | 1 mineral water                                  | 0      | 0   |
| 9.35  | 1 cup herbal tea                                 | 15     | 0   |
|       | Total                                            | 10 380 | 69.7 |

Julia actually considered that she ate a very healthy diet and was shocked to discover how much fat she was eating. She had seriously underestimated the fat content of such foods as lecithin granules (11g per tablespoon), macadamia nuts, health food bars and mayonnaise. Her total fat consumption was well above the recommended daily allowance.

*Nikki, aged 39. Young mum with two preschool children.*

|  |  | kJ | Fat |
|---|---|---|---|
| 5.30 | 1 cup white tea | 55 | 1 |
|  | 1 gingernut biscuit | 170 | 1 |
| 7.30 | 1/2 cup oatbran and fruit cereal | 530 | 2.5 |
|  | 1 slice toast, butter and Vegemite | 543 | 7 |
|  | 1 white tea | 55 | 1 |
| 9.30 | 1/2 apple | 135 | 0 |
| 10.10 | 1 white tea | 55 | 1 |
|  | 1 chocolate Tim Tam | 985 | 13 |
| 12.35 | 1/2 peanut butter and banana sandwich | 1670 | 25 |
|  | 1/4 date and banana sandwich | 366 | 3.5 |
|  | 1 ham and salad sandwich | 1255 | 17 |
|  | 200ml apple juice | 390 | 0 |
| 2.50 | 1/2 peach | 82 | 0 |
| 3.20 | 1 white tea | 55 | 1 |
|  | 1 chocolate Tim Tam | 985 | 13 |
| 5.30 | 1/4 cup tuna mornay | 835 | 12 |
|  | 1/2 slice brown bread and butter | 280 | 4.5 |
| 7.00 | 1 glass white wine | 375 | 0 |
| 8.00 | 1 serve cottage pie with peas and carrots | 2385 | 36 |
|  | 1 glass white wine | 375 | 0 |
|  | Total | 11 581 | 138.5 |

Nikki was staggered at the amount of fat she was consuming and admitted that her downfall was eating the children's leftovers—somehow she just couldn't bring herself to throw food out. Also, she seriously underestimated the amount of kilojoules and fat in foods such as chocolate biscuits.

## Tony, 52. Crane driver with a moderately active lifestyle.

| | | kJ | Fat |
|---|---|---|---|
| 6.30 | 1 white tea with 2 teaspoons sugar | 225 | 1 |
| 7.30 | 1 bacon and egg muffin | 1585 | 20 |
| | 1 hash brown | 545 | 7 |
| | 1 orange juice | 300 | 1 |
| | 1 white coffee with 2 teaspoons sugar | 275 | 1.5 |
| 11.00 | 1 white tea with 2 teaspoons sugar | 225 | 1 |
| | 1 Vegemite sandwich | 1985 | 14 |
| 1.15 | 1 roast beef and pickle sandwich | 1920 | 23 |
| | 1 malted milkshake | 1465 | 12 |
| 4.0 | 1 regular French fries | 1775 | 23 |
| 5.40 | 1 middy beer | 440 | 0 |
| | 30g peanuts | 795 | 16 |
| 6.10 | 1 middy beer | 440 | 0 |
| 8.00 | 2 spring rolls | 840 | 10 |
| | 1 bowl crab and corn soup | 670 | 4 |
| | 1 serve chicken chow mein | 1630 | 26 |
| | 1 cup fried rice | 1500 | 14 |
| | 2 × 375ml bottles beer | 1200 | 0 |
| 10.25 | 1 white tea with 2 teaspoons sugar | 225 | 1 |
| | Total | 18 040 | 174.5 |

Tony had a classic beer belly but insisted that he ate well and didn't drink too much—that was before I asked him to keep a food diary. After analysing the kilojoule and fat content of his average day he was determined to improve his diet. With nearly 175g of fat a day, it was no wonder that he was rotund.

---

So the first step in successful fat loss is to keep a food diary for 1 week. Don't change the way you eat at all. Simply note down everything you eat and drink then calculate the kilojoule and fat content. This may seem to be taking up a lot of time before you get started on your new eating plan, but it is important to see where your extra kilojoules have come from so that you can make better food choices and/or any lifestyle changes necessary for the program.

Whatever your reason for wanting to reduce body fat (and I say that rather than 'to lose weight', because that is what we are trying to achieve), you'll find strategies in this book that will successfully outsmart your fat cells, allow you to shrink them without triggering the famine response and hopefully lead you on an enjoyable journey, full of good food, fun and renewed vitality. Following the path I've outlined you can coax your body into a slimmer, healthier state. You *will* lose body fat, which *will* slim you down; you *will* regain a more youthful shape and have more energy for the good things in life. It's a path well worth taking with fine rewards along the way.

---

### Average daily energy consumption to maintain mean body weight:

*Women of 60kg body weight:*
18–35 years = 8400kJ 2000Cals
36–54 years = 7600kJ 1800Cals
55 plus = 6400kJ 1525Cals
Add or subtract approximately 400kJ (95Cals) for every 5kg above or below 60kg body weight.

*Men of 75kg body weight:*
18–35 years = 12 200kJ 2900Cals
36–54 years = 11 150kJ 2650Cals
55 plus = 9425kJ 2244Cals
Add or subtract approximately 600kJ (145Cals) for every 5kg above or below 75kg body weight.

---

# 4 Nutrition and weight loss

When you set out to reduce body fat, it's important to understand the role nutrition plays in weight gain and weight reduction. To most of us these days, food is pure pleasure—it's a reward, a comfort, a joy. But how many of us actually pay any attention to the real reason we've been given an appetite—nourishment. I can hear the howls of protest now:

*'I don't want to think of how good something is for me, I just want to enjoy it.'*
*'Food is the only thing left I don't have to worry about.'*
*'I simply don't have time to worry about the food I eat.'*

But if you seriously want to lose that excess fat forever, it's important to invest a little time in understanding how food works in our bodies. By doing some thoughtful preparation before adopting your new way of eating—which you'll love—you won't have to think about it any more because it will become natural to you.

Understanding how our bodies work and what they need to function properly is more than half the battle in regaining a natural body size. So let's go back to basics for a moment.

The reason we eat is to provide our bodies with water, carbohydrate, fats, protein, vitamins, minerals and trace elements to maintain it in peak condition. These nutrients have to be supplied in proper proportion to each other to maintain optimum health.

It's not necessary for us to measure and weigh, calculate and adjust all these elements, because Mother Nature has done this for us in natural foods. As long as we eat a wide variety of the foods that are in season we gain all the nourishment we need in the correct proportions. However, few of us these days follow a natural pattern of eating. Much of our food is highly processed. In refining foods most of the nutrients are stripped away and, even though some are then replaced, much of what we consume bears little relationship to the natural balance of nutrients we need every day for health. Even when we buy raw ingredients we cook most of them, which destroys a large percentage of the vitamin content and leaches away many of the minerals. Many of us eat very little raw food, if any.

Lack of dietary fibre and increased consumption of fat, vitamin and mineral deficiencies cause major imbalances in the way our bodies function. Many of these imbalances affect the way fat is metabolised and stored. It's not just from overeating, or eating too much fat, that we gain fat deposits over the years.

For example, for fat to be used as a fuel your body requires energy to metabolise it. The B vitamins, especially B6, are vital for this energy production, so that if your diet is lacking in these vitamins your body may not be able to burn fat efficiently. The rate of fat burning is also greatly reduced if your body doesn't have enough pantothenic acid and protein.

Energy for fat burning is produced by many enzymes which need a good supply of protein to function efficiently. If your diet is low in protein these enzymes are unable to do their job. To be efficiently used by these enzymes, protein itself needs the presence of many other nutrients such as choline and vitamin B6.

A deficiency in vitamin E can also slow fat metabolism, while a good supply of this vitamin will almost double our fat-burning capacity. Lecithin is another nutrient which helps the body to burn fat. If there is any deficiency in the nutrients necessary for lecithin production, especially choline and inosital, then our fat-burning capacity is lowered again.

So you see, by understanding what constitutes a 'well-balanced diet' you can maximise your body's fat-burning potential while increasing your health and vitality. It's not just a matter of popping a few vitamin pills, however. Nature has provided us with the best nutrients in whole foods. Studies have shown that when people adopt a wide-ranging whole food diet, their health improves dramatically compared with others who eat a normal Western diet with vitamin and mineral supplements. It seems that Nature has not yet revealed all the nutritive secrets of 'real' food.

By eating a wide variety of unrefined food you will give your body all the nutrients you need to keep your system in perfect balance and good working order. This not only keeps you healthy but also slows the ageing process. Refined foods do none of these things, while indiscriminate use of vitamin and mineral supplements can do more harm than good—increasing the amount of one nutrient may actually cause a deficiency in another. For example, if you take high amounts of zinc, perhaps to help a skin complaint, this may interfere with your body's use of copper, which in turn may cause incomplete iron metabolisation. In addition, when you add zinc to the diet you also need larger amounts of vitamin A. So popping a few pills that you buy at the supermarket will not necessarily help your health or vitality. Eating well will.

To normalise body fat levels, boost energy, reduce stress and give you a greater sense of well-being, it's important to look at what you eat as well as the amount of food you consume, and to plan a sensible, long-range eating plan that you'll love, which by its very nature will include all essential nutrients.

It's not in the scope of this book to cover every aspect of nutrition, which is a subject in itself, but below I look at those nutrients which are essential for maintaining health and vitality while on a fat-reducing program. Nutrients which may be beneficial in fat reduction include vitamin B complex, vitamin B2, vitamin B6, vitamin B12, choline, folic acid, inositol, pantothenic acid, vitamin C, vitamin E, calcium, manganese, magnesium, phosphorus, and unsaturated fatty acids (yes, even on a fat-loss diet you need some fats to achieve fat loss and to stay healthy).

## Vitamin B complex

The group of vitamins known as the B complex helps the body to produce energy from food by aiding the conversion of carbohydrate to glucose—the body's main fuel. The B complex vitamins include B1 (thiamine), B2 (riboflavin), B3 (niacin), B5 (pantothenic acid), B6 (pyridoxine), B12 (cyanocobalamin), B15 (pangamic acid), biotin, choline, folic acids, inositol, and para-amniobenzoic acid (PABA).

The presence of these vitamins in the body is vital to the metabolism of both fats and proteins. They are also essential for a well-functioning liver and gastrointestinal tract, the nervous system, and for maintaining healthy skin, hair and eyes.

Good sources of the B-group vitamins are brewer's yeast (the richest source), liver, wholegrain cereals, pulses, milk and milk products, eggs, meat, avocado (an excellent source of B6), bananas (an excellent source of B6), fish (an excellent source of B6 and B12), and wheat germ, green vegetables and nuts (good sources of folic acid).

## Vitamin C

Also known as ascorbic acid, vitamin C acts like the conductor of the orchestra—its presence is required to keep almost all systems working properly. Its functions include:

- aiding the metabolism of the amino acids, phenylalanine and tyrosine
- production and maintenance of collagen, a protein required for connective tissue in bones, ligaments and skin
- acting as a free radical scavenger
- helping detoxify the body of certain drugs and metabolic waste products
- helping to heal wounds and burns
- fighting bacterial infection
- improving the body's ability to absorb iron.

Without regular supplies of vitamin C the body is battling to perform most of its biological functions, including proper digestion and fat metabolism.

Good sources of vitamin C are most fruits and vegetables (guava, rockmelon, strawberries, kiwifruit, Brussels sprouts, capsicum and tomatoes being particularly rich sources).

> To keep your body constantly supplied with vitamin C it is important to eat vitamin C-rich foods with every meal. Vitamin C reaches its maximum level in the bloodstream about 2–3 hours after having been consumed. It is then quickly used up and what remains is excreted in the urine and through perspiration. The body has no mechanism for storing vitamin C. All vitamin C is either used up or eliminated about 4 hours after it has been ingested. Taking a large dose, such as a 1000mg tablet, at any one time is simply wasted, as most of it will be excreted in your urine. It is much better to take smaller doses, through eating fruit and vegetables, throughout the day.

## Vitamin E

Vitamin E is a fat-soluble vitamin which plays an essential role in the overall well-being. Its functions include:

- maintaining healthy heart, muscles and skeletal tissue
- nourishment of cells
- strengthening of the capillary walls and protection of red blood cells
- acting as an antioxidant by preventing saturated fatty acids from breaking down and combining with other substances harmful to the body
- helping to prevent premature ageing of the skin and maintain elasticity of the skin as you lose body fat.

Good sources of vitamin E include brans and legumes (especially wheat germ and soya beans), nuts, seeds and oils (especially wheat germ oil).

## Calcium

We all know that calcium is necessary for healthy teeth and bones, but calcium plays a far greater role in our well-being than that. Its functions include:

- producing energy and movement
- maintaining strong muscles

- acting as a natural tranquilliser, which keeps our nervous system in good working order
- helping to keep our skin young and healthy.

Calcium is not easily absorbed by the body—only about 20–30 per cent of dietary calcium is utilised and to facilitate its absorption other nutrients, such as vitamins A, C and D, magnesium and phosphorus have to be present. A certain amount of fat moving slowly through the digestive tract is also important for proper calcium absorption—which is another reason for including small amounts of unsaturated fat in your diet. However, when too much fat is eaten it combines with calcium to form an insoluble solution which can't be absorbed by the body.

It's best to eat calcium-rich foods at different times from iron-rich food because calcium can reduce the absorption of iron by the body. For example, have a low-fat yoghurt as a mid-morning or mid-afternoon snack, instead of eating it with a main meal which includes iron rich foods such as meat. If you're taking a calcium supplement, it's more easily absorbed at night, so take it just before bedtime—one benefit of this is that it will help you get a good night's sleep.

Good sources of calcium include low-fat, calcium-enriched milk products, low-fat, calcium-enriched soy products, low-fat cheeses, canned fish with edible bones (like salmon and sardines), tofu and tempeh, green vegetables, such as broccoli, and dried beans.

# Iron

Iron is one of the minerals essential for oxygen transportation around the body, especially to the brain, which requires a good supply of oxygen to function properly. If you're lacking iron, you may find it difficult to concentrate, remember or learn things. If your body is low in iron you'll also be prone to illness, because the cells which fight infection depend on adequate stores of iron to function efficiently. Iron is also essential for producing energy, so if you have an iron deficiency you will feel tired, lethargic and lacking vitality.

The best way to avoid an iron deficiency is to eat iron-rich food 4–5 times a week. Best sources of iron include lean beef, lamb and liver; medium sources include pork, chicken and fish. Some pulses and vegetables contain iron but it's not as easily absorbed by the body as iron from meat.

If you are a vegetarian and depend on plant foods for your iron, then make sure you include a vitamin C-rich food in the same meal to help the body absorb this type of iron.

## Magnesium

Magnesium is essential to the proper functioning of nerves and muscles, including the heart, and to many metabolic processes in the body, especially the utilisation of carbohydrates and amino acids. It helps promote the absorption of other vitamins and minerals such as vitamin B complex, vitamins C and E, calcium, sodium, potassium and phosphorus.

Magnesium is found mainly in green leafy vegetables. Other sources include raw, unmilled wheat germ, soy beans, milk, whole grains, seafood, figs, corn, apples and oil-rich seeds and nuts, especially almonds.

It's important to eat some of these foods in the natural raw state as processing and cooking leaches out magnesium.

## Manganese

Manganese is a trace mineral which acts as a catalyst in the synthesis of fatty acids and cholesterol. It's essential for the production of thyroxine, a hormone secreted from the thyroid gland, which helps control the body's metabolic rate. Deficiencies in thyroxine can lead to symptoms such as weight gain and fatigue, among others. Manganese is also essential to maintain healthy bones, help nourish the brain and nervous system, and maintain a proper balance in the production of sex hormones.

Good sources of manganese include wholegrain cereals, egg yolks, nut, seeds, and green vegetables.

## Phosphorus

Phosphorus is vital for the proper metabolism of fats, carbohydrates and proteins. For example, phospholipids such as lecithin help break up and transport fats and fatty acids around the body. Niacin and riboflavin can't be absorbed unless phosphorus is present. It is essential for the growth, maintenance and repair of cells and for the production of energy and also helps to keep the nervous system healthy and the brain functioning efficiently.

Good sources of phosphorus are meat, fish, poultry, whole grains, seeds and nuts.

## Unsaturated fatty acids (UFAs)

It's important to understand the role that fat plays in our well-being. We all need some fat in our diet to provide the essential fatty acids and fat-soluble vitamins—A, D, E and K—required for good health. However, we have to eat the right fats to achieve this.

The properties in fats which give them their characteristic flavour, texture and melting points are known as the 'fatty acids'; there are two main types—saturated fatty acids and unsaturated fatty acids.

Saturated fatty acids are usually solid at room temperature and usually come from animal sources, such as butter and the fat we see on meat.

Unsaturated fatty acids are usually liquid at room temperature and usually come from non-animal sources such as vegetables, seeds and nut oils. It's the unsaturated fats which have proven beneficial to our health.

The unsaturated fatty acids are further divided into two groups—the monounsaturates and polyunsaturates. To maintain our health no more than 25 per cent of our daily kilojoules should come from fats and these should be from the polyunsaturated or monounsaturated types.

Polyunsaturated fats are mainly found in vegetable oils (such as corn, safflower, sunflower, walnut, soybean), nuts, cereals and oily fish such as sardines, mackerel, tuna and salmon.

Monounsaturated fats are found in foods such as olives and olive oil, canola oil, macadamia nuts and oil, peanuts and peanut oil, and avocado.

## Quick guide to types of fat

| High in saturated fat | High in mono-unsaturated fat | High in poly-unsaturated fat |
|---|---|---|
| Butter, cooking margarine, lard | Monounsaturated margarine | Polyunsaturated margarine |
| Coconut oil, palm oil, palm kernel oil, soybeans | Monounsaturated oils, e.g. olive and canola oils | Polyunsaturated oils, e.g. sunflower and safflower oils |
| Meat fat, poultry skin | Nuts (peanuts, cashews and almonds), peanut butter | Nuts (walnuts, hazelnuts and brazil nuts) |
| Dairy fat—cheese, cream, icecream, yoghurt, full cream milk | Seeds | Seeds |
| | Avocado | |
| Commercial biscuits, cakes and pastries | | |
| Snack foods | | |
| Many takeaway foods | | |

# The omega fatty acids

There has been much talk in recent years about omega fatty acids and their effect on health. While there is no doubt that including omega-3 fatty acids in the diet in the form of fish such as tuna, mackerel, salmon, etc. is very beneficial to health, the same can't be said for omega-6 fatty acids. Let me explain. Omega-3 fatty acids are a class of long-chain polyunsaturated fats which differ in their chemical structure from the omega-6 polyunsaturated fatty acids found in vegetable oils and margarine. Recent research has shown that to maintain good health we need a balance between these fatty acids in our diet.

Over the last couple of decades there has been an increase of omega-6 fats in the Western diet, mainly due to people switching from butter to polyunsaturated oils and margarine. We now consume these fats in the ratio of about 50 parts omega-6 to 1 part omega-3. The ideal balance has been estimated to be in the region of 6:1 and to achieve this we need to eat less omega-6 and more omega-3 fats. Omega-3 fats have many health benefits including:

- preventing blood clots from forming
- preventing blockages of the arteries
- reducing triglyceride levels
- lowering LDL (bad) and raising HDL (good) cholesterol
- reducing blood pressure
- providing protection against cancer
- reducing joint stiffness and pain in rheumatoid arthritis
- reducing inflammation in skin conditions such as psoriasis.

All good reasons for including more fish in our diet.

---

### Fat-watching guide

**Vegetables**

*Good choices*
- All fresh, frozen, dried and tinned vegetables
- Salads
- Frozen mono- and polyunsaturated chips, oven-fried, which carry the Heart Foundation's Tick of Approval
- Dried beans and peas, e.g kidney beans, lentils and split peas
- Tinned beans, e.g baked beans, kidney beans, three bean mix

---

*Bad choices*
- Any vegetables with added fats, e.g in a butter sauce
- Takeaway chips
- Snack chips/crisps

**Fruits**
*Good choices*
- All fresh, tinned and dried fruits
- Fruit juices
- Fruit spreads
- Avocados and olives (in moderation)

*Bad choices*
- Coconut flesh, coconut cream and coconut milk

**Breads**
*Good choices*
- All types of breads, bread rolls, crumpets, English muffins, etc.
- Lebanese bread, pita bread, pocket bread, pumpernickel, sourdough
- Fruit bread, plain fruit buns
- Focaccia, bagels, baps, matzo, chapatti
- Crispbreads, crackerbread, rice cakes

*Bad choices*
- Breads made with added cheese and bacon
- Garlic bread
- Croissant
- Brioche

**Rice and pasta**
*Good choices*
- Brown rice
- White rice
- Wild rice
- Rice bran
- Rice cakes
- Pasta, wholemeal pasta

*Bad choices*
- Fried rice
- Commercial pasta dishes

## Grains and cereals

*Good choices*

- Wheat, rye, oats, barley, millet, bulgur, buckwheat, couscous, polenta
- Oat bran, barley bran, wheat bran, wheat germ
- Low-fat breakfast cereals
- Natural (untoasted) muesli
- Porridge
- Flour—white, wholemeal, self-raising, unbleached, cornflour, arrowroot
- Sago, tapioca, semolina

*Bad choices*

- Commercial sweet biscuits, cakes, pastries and muffins
- Cheese biscuits
- Toasted muesli
- Toasted or oven-baked breakfast cereals

## Meat

*Good choices*

- Any raw meat trimmed of all visible fat
- Any cooked cold meat trimmed of all visible fat
- Low-fat mince
- Lean meat patties
- Any meat product which carries the Heart Foundation's Tick of Approval

*Bad choices*

- Fatty meats
- Meat with visible fats
- Offal
- Tinned meat products
- Paté
- Meat pies, sausage rolls, hot dogs, etc.
- Fatty bacon
- Ordinary sausages
- Fatty cold meats—devon, salami, etc.

## Poultry

*Good choices*

- Chicken with skin and fat removed

- Turkey with skin and fat removed
- Duck with skin and fat removed

*Bad choices*

- Fried chicken
- Chicken which has been crumbed or battered
- Processed chicken products—pressed chicken, nuggets, etc.
- Takeaway chicken (other than skinless barbecued)

## Fish

*Good choices*

- All fresh fish
- Fish canned in brine or spring water, i.e. salmon, tuna, mackerel, sardines, etc.
- Smoked fish
- Frozen fish products which carry the Heart Foundation's Tick of Approval

*Bad choices*

- Fish in batter
- Regular fish fingers
- Frozen fish meals

## Seafood

*Good choices*

- Mussels
- Oysters
- Scallops
- Abalone
- Crabs
- Clams
- Lobster
- Crayfish
- Yabbies
- Marron
- Balmain and Moreton Bay bugs
- Prawns
- Calamari, squid, octopus
- Canned seafood, i.e. crab, prawns, etc.

*Bad choices*

- Any seafood in batter, crumbs or with cheese or cream sauces

**Dairy products**
*Good choices*
- Any reduced or low-fat milk
- Calcium-enriched milks
- Reduced-fat flavoured milk
- Low-fat yoghurt
- Low-fat cheese—ricotta, cottage, quark (fat content must be below 10%)
- Low-fat icecream
- Sorbets
- Frozen low-fat yoghurt
- Fruit-based gelati
- Fat-free fruit confections

*Bad choices*
- Full-cream or regular milk (liquid and powder)
- Goat's milk
- Full-cream flavoured milk
- Full-cream and regular yoghurt
- Regular cheese
- Commercial dips
- Regular icecream
- Cream, sour cream, lite sour cream, reduced cream and thickened cream
- Butter of all types

**Eggs**
*Good choices* (Note: don't have more than 2–3 eggs a week)
- Poached or boiled eggs
- Egg substitutes, i.e. Scramblers™ and Ready Eggs™
- Egg whites

*Bad choices*
- Fried eggs
- Mayonnaise
- Sauces made with eggs such as hollandaise or bearnaise

**Seeds, nuts and nut products**
*Good choices*
- Small amounts of all natural and dry roasted nuts and seeds

*Bad choices*
- Oil-roasted nuts
- Chocolate-coated nuts
- Peanut butter, tahini or other seed pastes
- Deep fried nuts

**Pastries**
*Good choices*
- Filo
- Pizza bases

*Bad choices*
- Shortcrust, puff, wholemeal
- Pies, pastries
- Danish pastries and croissants

**Fats and oils**
*Good choices*
- Small amounts of olive or canola oil
- Small amounts of reduced-fat spreads with the Heart Foundation's Tick of Approval

*Bad choices*
- Oils such as palm, palm kernel, coconut oil
- Hydrogenated vegetable oils
- Solid vegetable frying fats
- Commercial vegetable oils
- Blended vegetable oils
- Cooking margarine
- Butter, dairy blends
- Lard, dripping, ghee
- Suet
- Copha
- Any spread which doesn't carry the Heart Foundation's Tick of Approval

**Salad dressings**
*Good choices*
- Small amounts of olive or canola oil
- Low-joule salad dressings
- No-oil salad dressings
- Fat-free mayonnaise which carries the Heart Foundation's Tick of Approval
- Vinegars, lemon and lime juice

*Bad choices*
- Any cream-based dressing
- Sour cream dressings
- Cheese-style dressings, i.e blue vein, etc.
- Mayonnaise
- Ranch-style dressings

**Sauces**

*Good choices*
- Sauces such as tomato, barbecue, soy, mustard, Worcestershire, chilli or horseradish
- Tomato-based pasta sauces
- Fruit sauces such as apple, cranberry, etc.
- Commercial gravy powder
- Chutneys

*Bad choices*
- Butter and cheese sauces
- Cream sauces, i.e. bechamel, etc.
- Gravy made from meat fats

**Beverages**

*Good choices*
- Water, plain or mineral
- Low-joule soft drinks
- Cordials
- Tea, coffee and substitutes
- Fruit and vegetable juices
- Light soy drinks

*Bad choices*
- Coffee whiteners
- Milk shakes, thick shakes, etc.
- Whole flavoured milk
- Alcohol

**Takeaways**

*Good choices*
- Sandwiches, bread rolls, pita bread with low-fat fillings
- Salads with low-fat dressing
- Low-fat yoghurts
- Fresh fruit and fruit salad

- Baked potatoes with low-fat toppings
- Steamed rice and stir-fried vegetables
- Skinless chicken
- Lean meat kebabs
- Corn on the cob
- Burritos with beans and salad
- Low-fat steamed dim sims

*Bad choices*
- Fried and battered foods
- Meat pies, sausage rolls, chiko rolls, pluto pups, hot dogs
- Potato scallops, potato cakes, hash browns
- Pizza
- Fried rice
- Fatty chicken, fried and battered chicken, chicken nuggets
- Commercial hamburgers and cheeseburgers
- Hot chips, French fries
- Fried dim sims and spring rolls
- Any deep-fried Asian dishes or those containing coconut milk/cream

**Snacks**
*Good choices*
- Low-fat yoghurt
- Fresh and dried fruit
- Raw vegetable sticks with low-fat yoghurt
- Fruit bars (made from all fruit)
- Popcorn (microwaved or air popped, no butter)
- Crispbreads and rice cakes

*Bad choices*
- Biscuits
- Chocolate
- Potato crisps, corn chips, soy chips
- Extruded snack products i.e. Twisties, Cheezels, etc.
- Muesli bars
- Cakes

# 5  Exercise and fat loss

Any successful fat-loss program has to include exercise and it's important to understand why, so that you become committed to including it in your lifestyle. In earlier chapters I explained how the body will do everything it can to hoard and retain its fat, which may make it seem an impossible task to reverse it. However, there is a simple key to making the body unlock its fat stores—it's through exercise—and we can do it in three ways.

Firstly, exercise burns kilojoules, which helps use up the food we've eaten. At first the body will use carbohydrates as its primary fuel, but after a certain time, usually about 30–40 minutes, it will start to burn fat. If your diet doesn't have a high fat content then your body will start to use fat from its stores, and slowly over time your body fat will reduce.

Secondly, muscle requires energy for maintenance and movement. Muscle burns kilojoules even when you're in bed asleep at night—fat doesn't. So the more muscle your body has the more kilojoules it takes to maintain your basic metabolic rate.

Thirdly, as muscle mass increases and is used more, your body makes greater amounts of the lipolytic (fat-releasing) enzymes, so that when you exercise fat is released more easily.

Now I'm not suggesting that you become a weightlifter and develop bulging pecs and lats. In fact, for unfit fat people this activity would not be as effective in burning fat as moderate intensity, long duration walking. What I mean is that simply getting your muscles into good working order, so that they are strong and well-toned, will achieve the results you want. Your body fat will decline, you'll feel fitter, have more energy and look younger too.

It's important not only to increase your 'planned' level of exercise but also the 'incidental' activities in your day. It really is important to be as active as possible. If you can walk to the shops instead of driving the car, do so. Wash the car yourself rather than go to a drive-through car wash; climb stairs instead of taking the lift; play footy/cricket with your kids. Do everything which will make you get out of that seat and move around. The amount of energy used for each activity may be relatively small but it all adds up to a significant amount throughout the day.

The good news about exercise and fat burning is that you have to start slowly and build up—so don't feel you have to begin running 10 kilometres a day or doing heavy bench-presses to achieve results. You're retraining your body and for maximum effect this has to be done steadily over a period of time. After all, it has taken years for your body to get to this state and it's going to take some time to reverse it. However, you'll start to see results in just a few weeks!

Studies have shown that optimum fat burning in unfit, overweight people occurs at a lower exercise intensity level than that required for slim, fit people. And they will burn more fat if they exercise for longer at a lower intensity than if they exercise for a shorter period at a higher intensity. So your fat-loss exercise plan should start with long, low to medium intensity aerobic activities, such as walking, jogging or beginner aerobics. Over time, as your body adapts and you become stronger and fitter, you can slowly increase the intensity. Keeping an exercise chart is a good way of setting and reaching your exercise goals while encouraging you to stick to your program.

## Good fat-burning exercises

### WALKING

Walking is one of the best exercises for overall fitness and weight control because it uses almost all of the body's muscles and is especially good for the major muscles of the upper and lower legs, the buttocks, back and abdomen. It also gives your whole body a good aerobic workout.

### JOGGING

Jogging is one of the most effective fat-burning activities, and some people can become quite addicted to it. However, it is often uncomfortable for overweight people and can cause knee and ankle injuries. Many people are better off starting with walking to lose weight and build up muscles before turning to jogging. If, however, you do decide that jogging is for you, then make sure you get yourself some good jogging shoes to cushion your joints against the impact of running on hard surfaces.

### AEROBICS

Joining an aerobics class can be good fun and effective for burning fat. These classes are sociable, use lots of energy and promote muscle tone as well as fat loss. Make sure you begin in a class which is suitable for your level of fitness. Remember, the best fat loss comes initially from long duration, low to medium intensity exercise. If you join an advanced class you'll not only risk injury but won't achieve the best results.

### CYCLING

Cycling is good for building up the major muscles in your legs but doesn't do much for the upper body. However, if you include cycling as part of a weekly exercise program including walking, aerobics etc. it can be enjoyable and effective. On the bike make use of the 'easy' gears, to increase the aerobic benefit and reduce the chance of knee pain.

## STRENGTH TRAINING

Strength training involves the use of weights to exercise isolated muscles or groups of muscles. This is not recommended for the start of your fat-loss program but is a useful addition once your fitness improves and your body adapts to the level of activity you've achieved. To gain best results and avoid injury it's advisable to work out under the supervision of a properly qualified instructor.

## EXERCISE COMBINATIONS

To maximise the benefits of your fat-burning exercise it's a good idea to do different exercises over the course of the week. This not only maintains your interest but makes sure that all your muscles are given a good workout. A program that includes walking, aerobics, cycling, strength training, aquarobics and swimming will provide a total body workout, improve cardiovascular fitness, improve muscle tone, increase flexibility and burn that fat.

When you first start to exercise you may feel tired afterwards, but you'll probably sleep better at night and wake more refreshed next morning. As your program progresses your body will adapt to that amount of exercise and it will become easier for you to complete. This is when you should increase the pace and/or duration of the exercise. Slowly but surely your muscles will strengthen and enlarge; they'll start to produce more lypolitic enzymes for fat burning; and because muscles need energy (remember fat doesn't), your metabolism will be running at a higher rate.

---

### Monitoring your success

Your bathroom scales may not give a true indication of your changing body shape, especially if you are increasing muscle tone and size through exercise. The best way to monitor your size reduction is by keeping measurement charts. When you start your Fat-loss Eating Plan, take a note of your overall body measurements. Measure yourself once a week on the same day and note the changes on a chart. It will surprise you just how quickly you'll see results.

---

# 6 Strategies for reducing body fat

To successfully lose excess body fat, and keep it off permanently, we have to understand how our physiology works on a daily basis. Throughout each 24 hour period, our bodies follow a natural cycle called the circadian rhythm. As we wake and become active our metabolic rate increases and our body starts to look for fuel for the day's activities ahead. When we eat breakfast our metabolic rate is boosted further; it continues to climb through the morning to midday, when it plateaus, before starting to fall in the late afternoon and early evening in preparation for a night of sleep, when our metabolic rate is at its lowest. So our body's greatest need for food as fuel is first thing in the morning after the night's fast and also through the day when we are active. The time it doesn't require a lot of fuel is when it is preparing itself for, and during, sleep.

These days most of us eat in a reverse pattern to our body's actual need for food. We have a light breakfast, maybe just a bowl of cereal, then a sandwich and a drink for lunch, taking in our greatest number of kilojoules in the evening, when we sit down to a full dinner. This means we deprive the body of what it needs during the day, and give it what it doesn't need at night—it's no wonder that all the body can do with those extra kilojoules at night is store them.

So if you want to lose that extra fat, it's vital to adopt a more natural eating pattern—one which is biologically right for you. I can just hear all the objections:

*'I just can't eat breakfast.'*
*'I've no time to cook in the morning.'*
*'You try getting three kids off to school and worrying about nutrition—our house is bedlam in the morning!'*

But as I've said before in this book—your current body shape is the result of your present lifestyle and if you want to lose that fat, you are going to have to make some changes to the way you do things.

The good news is that there are some big payoffs from making just a few small adjustments in the way you eat. By adopting the Fat-loss Eating Plan outlined in Chapter 7, you'll:

- shed that extra fat and keep it off permanently
- find you have more energy throughout the day, which will help you

cope with your job, commuting, children, and home responsibilities far better than before.

There will also be a cascade of benefits:

- because you'll have more energy, you'll feel less stressed
- because you'll feel less stressed, you'll feel more motivated
- because you'll feel more motivated, you'll do more and get more out of life.

Isn't that worth trying even for a few weeks? I guarantee you'll look better, have better quality of sleep and feel much happier in yourself than you did before.

Now some people have told me that if they eat breakfast, they're starving again by 10.30am, but that if they skip breakfast they can go through until lunchtime without eating (the thinking being that this way they are cutting down on their daily kilojoules and will thus lose weight). Well, of course if they eat breakfast they will feel hungry again by 10.30am, because by providing the body with fuel first thing in the morning they've revved up their metabolism, which is now burning fuel at a higher rate.

In this Fat-loss Eating Plan you'll be eating again at 10.30am anyway, so hunger is never going to be a problem.

## Energy boosting/calming foods

Being able to tailor your mood to your activity can actually help you stick to your eating plan, because it reduces stress and allows you to cope with tasks more easily. For example, if you've felt tired and lethargic all day, every task will have seemed a chore, it will have taken an effort of will to get through the day, and you'll probably get home in the evening looking for a reward of some kind—usually in the form of comfort food and alcohol. It was a tough day, but you got through it, you deserve a treat, you can start over tomorrow.

On the other hand, if you've sailed through the day with lots of energy, and achieved all you've set out to, you'll feel pleased and satisfied with yourself. Consequently, you'll be far more likely to stick to your eating plan in the evening.

If you eat protein it will give you energy and drive—that's why I recommend eating protein for breakfast and lunch, when you want to be firing on all cylinders. Carbohydrates have a sedating effect on both mind and body—they boost our levels of serotonin, a neurotransmitter known to have a calming effect on the brain. Carbohydrates eaten in the evening will help you relax and unwind after a busy day.

The simple rule to remember is: *protein provides power, carbohydrate calms*. Most of us, however, eat these foods in reverse, having carbohydrates for breakfast and lunch and protein in the evening.

---

### Cheerful chilli

If you feel down-in-the dumps, instead of wolfing down a chocolate bar try a dish like Thai chilli chicken, Indian beef curry or a hot chilli con carne. Yes, that's right, chilli can lift your mood and give you a pleasurable high. You see, hot chillies contain a substance called capsaicin which causes the fiery sensation in your mouth. This reaction triggers the release of endorphins, natural painkillers, in the brain, which make you feel good. It's why chilli is one of the most popular spices in the world today.

---

## Eating properly

Whenever you eat a meal take the time to enjoy every mouthful of it without any distractions such as reading a book or watching television. Such distractions cause you to swallow your food and finish a meal without your brain consciously registering the pleasure of its flavour or the amount that you've eaten. When you've finished, your stomach is full but because your brain doesn't recognise this fact you may be tempted to go back for seconds or have a second or third course. The one exception to this effect is eating around a table with family and friends. This activity has a subtle effect on the way we appreciate and enjoy food—you are gathered around the food, it's the focus of attention, people talk about the aromas and flavour, the talk is often about food in general. All this combines to stimulate our palates and digestive system. Our brains are tuned into our stomachs and register not only the pleasure of the food but the experience as a whole. It's the reason that communal eating has been so popular with people of all nationalities down through the ages.

## Eat more slowly

Many people overeat simply because they eat too quickly and swallow food before it is properly chewed. Eating too quickly is a symptom of today's lifestyle, where a meal is often sandwiched in between other activities—it's a question of getting it over with so that we can go on to the next thing we have or want to do. We also don't chew food as well as we should.

### Eat your greens—they'll keep you happy

They say 'we are what we eat'—well, this could easily be changed to 'our mood comes from what we munch'. If you find yourself depressed by modern life, anxious about the future, unable to cope with all the demands placed on you, ask yourself this question: 'Am I eating enough green leafy vegetables every day?' If the answer is no, this could be the reason for your mood. You see, green leafy vegetables are rich in folic acid, one of the B-group vitamins, which is responsible for keeping our nervous system in good working order.

Clinical studies in Canada have revealed that people with a good intake of folic acid are generally happy and cheerful, while those deficient in folic acid suffer from depression and anxiety. So make sure you eat your greens—like spinach, broccoli and bok choy—several times a week. Other foods rich in folic acid are chicken livers, bulgur wheat, okra, orange juice and red kidney beans.

Next time you're eating, pay attention when you want to swallow each mouthful. Is everything in your mouth pureed, or are there still lumps of unchewed, but softened, food that you are about to swallow? If this the case, then you are not chewing your food properly—and you are not alone. Next time you're eating out watch how other people eat. In most cases food goes into the mouth, is given four or five chews, then swallowed quickly, followed by the next mouthful of food.

Thoroughly chewing our food, so that what we swallow is liquid not solid, has several important functions:

- It allows our taste buds to register the maximum pleasure from it.
- It prepares the food for digestion. As we chew, enzymes are released from our salivary glands which start the digestive process so that the food is in the right condition to be processed by the stomach.
- It slows the eating process so that the stomach has the time, usually about 15–20 minutes, to register that it is full and send a signal to the brain that you should stop eating.

So, as part of the Fat-loss Eating Plan I'm going to ask you to take the time to chew your food properly—what you swallow should be liquid with no solids in it. Because the food stays in your mouth longer you'll get more satisfaction from its flavour and find that you'll feel satisfied without overeating.

# Dining out

One of the great pleasures of life in this country is our wonderful food and great restaurants. Eating out is part of our lifestyle and the good news is you don't have to stop just because you are on the Fat-loss Eating Plan. Most restaurants these days cater for their more health-conscious clients and in most cases there will be plenty of tempting low-fat items on the menu for you to choose from. If not, ask for advice from the staff. In most cases they'll be happy to accommodate you by preparing a low-fat dish or modifying a menu item to reduce its fat content. However, there can be a few pitfalls for the unwary. Here's a guide to keeping your dining out experience a healthy low-fat one.

## CHINESE RESTAURANTS

All those crispy little morsels like spring rolls and fritters are the real killers here, so avoid anything which has been dipped in batter and/or deep-fried. Choose seafood, chicken, meat or vegetable dishes that have been steamed or stir-fried and order boiled rather than fried rice.

## FRENCH RESTAURANTS

If there's a French term on the menu you don't understand ask the waiter to explain how the dish is cooked so you can judge whether it's high in fat or not. Stay away from anything 'à la creme', 'à la mode', 'à la greque', 'à la king' or 'à la reine' because they will contain either cream or oil, or both.

## GREEK RESTAURANTS

Greek cuisine uses a lot of olive oil, which is good for you but only in small amounts. Decline anything which is bathed in oil. Good choices are dishes like stuffed vine or cabbage leaves, grilled seafood, meat dishes like souvlaki, and Greek salad (but have the dressing served separately so you can control the amount used). Greek desserts are delicious and deadly because they are generally loaded with kilojoules—just enjoy the wonderful coffee instead.

## INDIAN RESTAURANTS

Indian cuisine includes wonderful vegetarian dishes, so choose from these as long as they're not deep-fried or made with ghee, which can send the kilojoule count soaring. Dhals, bean and seafood dishes are also good choices. Side dishes are generally low-fat, as are chapattis, which are cooked on a griddle. Avoid pappadums as they are usually cooked in oil.

## ITALIAN RESTAURANTS

Avoid pan-fried dishes or pasta sauces that are rich in cream and cheese and go for veal or chicken braised in wine, seafood cooked in fresh tomato sauce, roasts and grills cooked with fresh herbs. Parmesan cheese is served with many Italian dishes so ask for it to be added sparingly, or served separately so you can add your own.

## JAPANESE RESTAURANTS

Japanese food is generally low in fat as long as you avoid fried dishes like tempura, and other battered or crumbed dishes. Sushi and sashimi are excellent choices, as are grilled meals like yakitori and simmered dishes like shabu shabu.

## MEXICAN RESTAURANTS

Mexican food can be high in fat if the dish is loaded with sour cream, avocado and cheese. However, there is still plenty to choose from on a Mexican menu. Try tacos, tortillas, enchiladas and bean dishes, for example. Also check the serving sizes, which tend to be very generous. If a large plateful is put in front of you, you will be tempted to eat it all. If portions are large, ask if you can have an entree size or share a dish with your companion/s.

## THAI RESTAURANTS

In general, Thai food is low in fat except where coconut milk or cream is used (1/2 cup has 1840kJ/440Cals and 27g fat). Also avoid deep-fried entree dishes such as prawn toasts, seafood bundles and fish patties. Go for grilled satays, seafood salads or a stir-fried dish instead.

The following strategies may also help when dining out:

- As soon as the waiter arrives with the menus order a salad to nibble on while you're deciding what else to eat. It will take the edge off your hunger.
- Order small portions. If you are still hungry you can always order another dish or fill up with a salad.
- Listen to your body and eat only to the point where you feel comfortable.

- Instead of an entree and a main course, order two entrees.
- If you have an entree, skip dessert, or vice versa.

## Read food labels carefully

When buying packaged and processed foods always look for the nutrition table on the pack—if it doesn't have one it usually means the product is high in fat, salt and preservatives and the manufacturer doesn't want you to know what's in it. Most reputable brands carry a nutrition table.

Under the Australian National Food Authority Code of Practice, 'fat-free' means that a product can contain up to 0.15g of fat per 100g of food, which means that it is low in fat but isn't actually fat-free. Also under this code the words 'lite' or 'light' can actually refer to a product's colour or flavour and not its fat content. This must be stated somewhere on the label but it can be in tiny print.

Another misleading term is '95% fat-free'. If this figure is calculated by weight rather than kilojoules the product can actually have quite a high fat content. To take a simple example, a product that weighs 100 grams and consists of 95 grams water and 5 grams of fat could be said to be 95% fat-free—by weight. However, if the calculation is based on kilojoules it would be 100% fat! So be wary of any product making these types of claims.

# 7  The fat-loss eating plan

I've explained why it's important to shed excess body fat, and why dieting has made this so difficult for most of us to achieve. Now, here is the simple eating plan that will help you lose that fat and keep it off permanently.

As outlined earlier, to change your body composition, and therefore your shape and the way you look, you need to eat a proper diet, take regular exercise, have a positive mental attitude AND reduce the amount of fat in your diet. You have to create an energy deficit to force your body to draw on its fat stores, thereby shrinking the size of your fat cells. This can be done by:

- eating less
- exercising more
- increasing muscle bulk
- all of the above.

Simply eating less will achieve temporary weight loss, but this is likely to come from muscle tissue as well as fat, which will lower your metabolism and result in increased weight gain when you return to normal eating—which may, in fact, be at a lesser kilojoule intake than prior to your diet.

With exercise alone it's hard to achieve lasting results because, firstly, few of us have the time it would take to fit that much exercise into our day and secondly, exercise increases our appetite, encouraging us to consume the equivalent number of kilojoules we've just burned off.

Increasing muscle size is helpful because the more muscle you have, the more energy your body needs to maintain itself. But simply increasing muscle size is not going to counteract the lifestyle elements that have given rise to your problems with fat in the first place.

It is the fourth option, combining all three elements, which is the successful way to lose that fat and keep it off permanently.

Let's look at the food side first. To lose 500g (1 pound) of body fat a week you have to create a deficit of 14 700kJ (3500Cals)—that's 2100kJ (500Cals) a day. The best way to achieve this is to burn an extra 1050kJ (250Cals) through exercise and eat 1050kJ less in food. To burn 1050kJ a day you would have to do one of these things:

- power walk for 25 minutes
- swim continuously for 25 minutes
- weight train for 25 minutes

- box for 25 minutes
- climb stairs for 25 minutes
- do a 30 minute beginners aerobics class
- do a jazzercise class for 35 minutes
- play 35 minutes of basketball
- cycle for 1 hour
- garden for 1 hour

## Be a tortoise, not a hare

It's really important to make a commitment to losing your excess fat the same way you gained it—slowly. Aim for a loss of 250–500g ($\frac{1}{2}$–1 pound) a week. This may not seem very much, but a gradual loss doesn't trigger the body's starvation responses, which fight your attempts to shrink its fat cells.

A healthy diet should be made up from approximately:

- 60–75% complex carbohydrate (refined carbohydrates and concentrated sugars such as white flour, white sugar, honey, fruit juices and dried fruit should account for no more than 10% total calories)
- 15–25% fats—from mono- or polyunsaturated fats
- 10–15% protein

The carbohydrate should come from whole grains and cereals, pulses, fruits and vegetables. The fats should be in the form of fish and seafood, lean poultry and meats, fruits such as avocado, seeds and nuts (tiny amounts of olive and canola oil can also be included). Protein should come from fish and seafood, lean poultry and meat, pulses, seeds, nuts, low-fat dairy products and grains.

A 70kg man of average height, undertaking light work, would need the following daily food intake to maintain that weight:

| Food | grams/day | kJ/day | % total kilojoules |
|------|-----------|--------|--------------------|
| Carbohydrate | 370g | 6300kJ (1500Cals) | 63% |
| Protein | 70g | 1200kJ (285Cals) | 12% |
| Fat | 65g | 2500kJ (595Cals) | 25% |
| Total | 505g | 10 000kJ (2380Cals) | 100% |

A 55kg woman of average height, undertaking light work, would require the following daily food intake to maintain that weight:

| Food | grams/day | kJ/day | % total kilojoules |
|---|---|---|---|
| Carbohydrate | 303g | 5093kJ (1212Cals) | 63% |
| Protein | 36g | 611kJ (145Cals) | 12% |
| Fat | 33g | 1273kJ (303cals) | 25% |
| Total | 372g | 6977kJ (1660Cals) | 100% |

*Note:* The gram weights of these nutrients do not represent the total weight of food eaten, as they don't take into account the dietary fibre, water content or nutrients.

In most Western countries these proportions are all jumbled up, with a typical diet containing 50–60% fat, 30% protein and 20% complex carbohydrate.

## Returning to a natural way of eating

Eating for successful fat loss really means *reverting to a natural way of eating*, with the main bulk of your food coming from the complex carbohydrates and a minimum amount from protein and fat. This comes as quite a surprise to most people because they are used to having large amounts of protein and fat with carbohydrates as just accompaniments—think of the typical 'meat and three veg' meal where a steak can be falling off the sides of the plate and the vegetables hardly make an appearance. In the Fat-loss Eating Plan I want you to think of protein—meat, chicken, fish, seafood, nuts, beans, etc.—almost as flavouring rather than the main ingredient. This won't be hard if you enjoy Asian style cuisines because that is how those cuisines are constructed—lots of vegetables and a little meat or fish to go along with them—and look how tasty and satisfying those meals are.

The second way of returning to a natural way of eating is to *consume the bulk of your kilojoules during the day*, or at least before 6.00pm, when your body is looking for food and running at a higher metabolic rate.

On the Fat-loss Eating Plan it's important to rearrange the kilojoule balance of your day so that you eat the bulk of your food (including your protein) through the day, then have a light carbohydrate meal at night.

Ask yourself each evening, before you start preparing dinner, 'Am I really hungry?' For many people who have eaten well during the day the

---

### Dietary fibre

It's really important to eat food high in dietary fibre, if you are to succeed in losing fat and keeping it off permanently. Foods high in dietary fibre:

- take longer to chew which promotes a feeling of fullness, so the brain signals you to stop eating
- increase the amount of fat excreted in the faeces
- improve digestion by increasing the secretion of digestive hormones
- improve tolerance to glucose
- speed the transit time of food through the digestive tract so that fat has less time to be absorbed.

It's recommended that we all consume between 30–50g fibre each day.

---

answer is 'No', because their bodies are slowing down and not really looking for fuel. If this is the case, have some fruit or non-fat yoghurt and a large glass of water. Thirst can sometimes make you think you are hungry when in fact you are just a little dehydrated. Have a non-alcoholic drink, wait ten minutes and see if you are still hungry. If you are, eat something; if not, use the time you would have spent cooking doing something you enjoy, like reading a book, listening to music, playing with the children. Don't do a chore or watch television. A chore may make you want to reward yourself with food. Television has so many food commercials that it's almost impossible not to give into the autosuggestion that you should eat something.

This brings us to the final key to successful fat loss. *Listen to your body*. If it is telling you it's hungry, then feed it. If it's not hungry, then don't. Not eating when your body is telling you it wants food risks switching on the 'famine' response, which will sabotage all your attempts to shrink your fat cells. Eating just because the clock says it's meal time, when your body is not sending signals that it needs fuel, is simply giving your body food to store. Many of us are so used to ignoring the signals that our body sends that it comes as quite a surprise when we finally do tune in and discover how eloquent it is in communicating its needs. By responding to what it is telling you, you will quickly bring all your systems back into balance, with the greater sense of well-being that this brings.

Everyone has different lifestyles and food requirements, so it is not possible to cover every situation in one book. However, here is the basic model for you to build on.

# The Fat-loss Eating Plan

## STEP 1: BREAKFAST

The first important step in shedding excess fat is to eat breakfast. Even if you don't normally feel hungry first thing in the morning, try to have something because it will boost your metabolism and get it running at a higher level for most of the day. And it's important to include some protein in it, even if it is only skim milk with cereal (skim milk has 9g protein per 250ml and no fat) or a skim milk smoothie to boost your energy levels. Try:

- Baked beans on wholemeal toast (spread the toast with mustard instead of butter if you like)
- Multigrain toast spread with mustard and topped with avocado and melted low-fat cheese
- Boiled or poached egg on wholemeal toast (only 2–3 eggs per week)
- Lean ham and asparagus with melted low-fat cheese.

These are just a few quick, healthy, protein breakfasts; for more see Breakfast recipes, page 68.

## STEP 2: MID-MORNING SNACK

If you're hungry by mid-morning have a nourishing, low-fat, mid-morning snack such as:

- A skim milk cappuccino
- A piece of fruit
- Non-fat yoghurt
- Rice cakes with jam
- Vegetable sticks and some low-fat cottage cheese
- Small cone of frozen non-fat yoghurt.

These will quell any hunger pangs, give your body the energy boost it's looking for and also provide it with some essential nutrients.

## STEP 3: LUNCH

This is when you should have the balance of your protein for the day (also see Energy boosting/calming foods, page 42). Having a proper meal at lunchtime can present a challenge for many people, but a little lateral thinking and a small amount of planning can overcome any problems. If your workplace is in an industrial area where the only food outlets sell pie-and-chips or hamburgers, then try to take lunch from home.

Again, I can hear the protests: 'Who has time to do that!', but again I say, it only takes a little organisation to produce a healthy, satisfying lunch-to-go, and remember, full meals can exist between two slices of bread. Leftover roast or baked meats and vegetables from the weekend, chutney, grain mustard and salad between slices of crusty multigrain bread make a hearty, satisfying meal.

If you want hot food, buy one of those wide-neck thermos flasks which have separate compartments. Soups, casseroles, curries, bolognese sauces, mashed potato, rice and pasta can all be cooked at the weekend, frozen in individual portions, then thawed overnight, zapped in the microwave in the morning, placed separately into the compartments of the flask—and you have a hot, tasty meal for lunchtime. Take along a multigrain bread roll and some fruit and you'll have a meal your co-workers will be envious of.

Of course, if your workplace is surrounded by a variety of food outlets then you can make a healthy choice following the guidelines outlined in this book.

---

### Hold the butter! Hold the mayo! Hold the margarine!

There are many good, fat-free spreads you can use in a sandwich in place of butter, margarine or mayonnaise. If you're having a beef sandwich, for instance, spread the bread with a mustard of your choice, then fill with beef and salad; for lamb, try mint jelly and grain mustard; for chicken, try cranberry sauce and avocado; for pork, try apple sauce and mango chutney. The list of combinations is only limited by your imagination!

---

## STEP 4: MID-AFTERNOON SNACK

If you are hungry, have a similar snack to your morning break, with perhaps a herbal tea to pep you up (try basil, mace, lemon balm or rosehip).

## STEP 5: EATING IN THE EVENING

Now, because your body has been well-fed all day and your metabolism is slowing down in preparation for sleep, you may not actually feel all that hungry. Many people eat an evening meal because that's what they do in the evening, or because it's a reward for getting through the day. Try to tune into what your body needs. If you don't feel hungry, don't eat.

However, if you get home and are starving after a day's work, then make yourself a hearty carbohydrate meal. Avoid protein, which takes longer for your body to digest. Carbohydrate is also relaxing and has a sedative effect, which is more appropriate for unwinding at the end of the day and preparing for a good night's sleep. Try non-fat vegetable soup, pasta with a no-oil tomato and vegetable sauce, vegetarian risotto—even a bowl of homemade muesli with fresh fruit and non-fat yoghurt would be good (rolled oats are particularly calming).

## THE WEEKEND

If you enjoy entertaining or eating out with friends, try to swap dinner for lunch on these occasions. Not only will you have longer to linger over the meal, but your body will have a greater time to use up the kilojoules as fuel, rather than having a large amount of food to contend with when its metabolism is running at its lowest. And you can always go for a leisurely stroll in the afternoon which will help burn up those kilojoules even faster.

If you like socialising with friends in the evening, try non-eating activities like going to the theatre, seeing a band, dancing, catching a movie—anything which doesn't involve eating as its main activity.

---

### Easy ways to reduce fat in your diet

- only choose low-fat protein foods such as lean meat trimmed of all fat, chicken with the skin removed, skim milk and other low-fat dairy products
- shun fried foods, pastries, deli meats, snack foods, rich cakes and biscuits
- choose low-fat takeaway foods such as salad sandwiches or rolls; fruit; barbecued chicken (without skin) and lean hamburgers (without the egg) with lots of salad; fruit salads, etc.
- use low-fat cooking methods such as grilling, steaming, baking and stir-frying (see Cooking techniques, page 59)

---

> - use mustards, chutneys, thick fruit purees, jellies, jams, low-fat cream cheese or avocado as sandwich spreads, or spread poly-unsaturated margarine only very thinly
> - skim fat from the tops of soups and casseroles
> - avoid battered or crumbed foods
> - use low-fat yoghurt, lemon juice or vinegar as salad dressings instead of mayonnaise or salad oils

## Working out your energy requirements

To begin the eating plan you have to work out how many kilojoules are keeping you at your present weight. To do this you simply multiply your weight in kilograms by the amount of kilojoules required by your activity level:

1. Inactive—126kJ (30Cals)
2. Light physical activity—147kJ (35Cals)
3. Moderate physical activity—168kJ (40Cals)
4. Heavy physical activity—189kJ (45Cals)

For example, if you are 75kg and live a moderately active life then you would need 12 600kJ (3000Cals) a day to maintain that weight. Remember, if you want to lose 500g of body fat a week, you have to create an energy deficit of 2100kJ (500Cals) per day. You could either reduce your energy intake to 10 500kJ (2500Cals), or you could reduce your food intake by 1050kJ (250Cals) and expend the equivalent amount in extra activity.*

Once you have reach your target weight of, say, 70kg, a dietary intake of 11 760kJ (2800Cals) will keep you there—provided, of course, that your daily activity level remains the same. If you become more active you can increase the amount of food you eat; if you become less active you should reduce it. Whatever your energy intake, however, you should still stick to the percentages of carbohydrate, protein and fat outlined above.

The mistake that many people make when they decide to lose weight is to go straight onto a 5000kJ (1200Cals) a day diet, which has been promoted as the minimum safe level of kilojoule restriction. This could be a drop of maybe 8400kJ (2000Cals) from their normal eating patterns—more than half their energy intake. The size and suddenness of the drop in

---

* 1Cal = 4.1 kJ; 1 stone = 6.35 kg; 1 pound = 454g

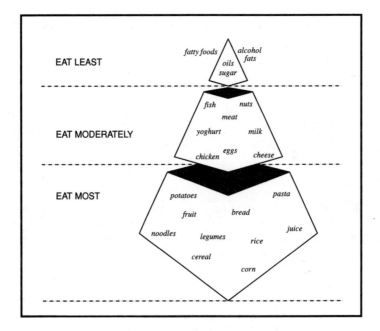

EAT LEAST

*fatty foods*  *alcohol*
*oils*  *fats*
*sugar*

EAT MODERATELY

*fish*  *nuts*
*meat*
*yoghurt*  *milk*
*chicken*  *eggs*  *cheese*

EAT MOST

*potatoes*  *pasta*
*fruit*  *bread*
*noodles*  *juice*
*legumes*  *rice*
*cereal*
*corn*

energy intake triggers all the famine responses in the body and they're almost defeated before they've begun. The only safe and effective way is to do it gradually, to fool your body into giving up its fat stores without it thinking it's under threat from famine.

# Eating from the five food groups

When planning your meals, simply make your choices from the five food groups according to the diet pyramid. The five food groups are:

## 1  BREADS AND CEREALS

Including fibre enriched white bread, multigrain and wholemeal; grains such as rice, oats and rye; pasta. These provide energy, fibre and B group vitamins.

- 4 or more servings a day
- 1 serving is equal to 1 slice of bread, 1/2 cup of cooked rice or pasta or 1 cup breakfast cereal.

## 2  FRUIT AND VEGETABLES

Rich in dietary fibre, they also provide B group vitamins, vitamins C and E, beta carotene (a powerful antioxidant) and potassium.

- 5 or more servings a day, including vitamin C-rich foods such as oranges, tomatoes, capsicum at each meal
- 1 serving of fruit is equal to 1 small apple, pear, mandarin, etc., 1/3 cup fruit juice, 12 grapes, 1/4 small rockmelon, 1 medium peach, 2 medium apricots, 1/2 cup pineapple chunks
- 1 serving of vegetables is equal to 1/2 cup raw or cooked vegetables, 1/3 cup corn kernels, 2/3 cup parsnips, 1 small potato, 1/2 cup mashed potato, 3/4 cup chopped pumpkin.

### 3  MEAT, FISH, POULTRY, EGGS, NUTS AND LEGUMES

This is the protein group which provides B-group vitamins including vitamin B12, and vital minerals such as iron and zinc.

- 1–2 servings a day
- 1 serving is equal to 100g cooked (180g raw) lean meat, fish or poultry, 1 egg, 1/4 cup nuts or 1/2–1 cup cooked peas, beans or lentils.

### 4  DAIRY PRODUCTS

Keep these to a minimum and only choose low-fat varieties of milk, cheeses, yoghurt, etc. Don't neglect your calcium intake and take a supplement if necessary.

- 1 serving a day
- 1 serving is equal to 1 cup non-fat milk, 1 cup non-fat yoghurt, 30g low-fat cheese.

### 5  FATS AND OILS

Try to keep these to a minimum and eat only fats from the following list:

- 4 serves a day
- 1 serve is equal to 1/8 of an avocado, 1 teaspoon olive or canola oil, 5 small olives, 10 whole almonds, 20 peanuts, 6 small nuts (walnuts, pecans, Brazils, hazel, etc.)

## How much fat is good for you?

In general, daily fat intake, which should be from mono- and polyunsaturated fat, should be no more than:

- children: 30–60g
- teenagers: 40–80g (provided they are active)
- women: 30–60g
- men: 40–80g
- labourers/athletes: 80–100g

# 8 Low-fat cooking techniques

Half the secret of reducing fat in your diet is changing to low-fat cooking techniques. This is no great hardship as they are no more labour-intensive than other methods, and you don't have to sacrifice any texture or flavour. For instance, just removing 2 tablespoons of fat from the frying or sauteeing process reduces the fat content of a dish by 40g!

## Barbecuing

Barbecuing is a great low-fat way of cooking. Whether you use an open wood fire, electric or gas barbecue or an enclosed kettle-style barbecue, the results will be mouthwateringly good. Heat your gas or electric barbecue to high. If using charcoal or wood allow the coals to die down until they turn white in daylight, or glowing red if cooking after dark. Here are some tips to get the best from your barbecue.

**Meat**
- Trim away any visible fat from meat and poultry to prevent flare-ups during cooking.
- Marinate the meat for anything from 30 minutes to overnight to add extra flavour and tenderise the meat.
- Seal meat on one side. When juices start to appear on the uncooked side, turn it over to seal other side. Continue cooking until done to taste.
- To test if meat is cooked to your liking, don't cut into it or pierce it with a fork because you'll lose tasty juices that way. Simply press the meat with tongs—if it feels springy, then it's rare. If it has a little resistance, then it's medium. Well done feels quite firm.

**Fish**
- Fillets and cutlets can be wrapped in foil parcels with lemon slices and cooked on top of the hot plate.
- If cooking directly on the hot plate, spray it with canola oil so that the fish doesn't stick to the metal surface.
- When cooking fish it's best to use medium to high heat on an electric barbecue, glowing embers on a wood or charcoal barbecue, and a medium flame on a gas barbecue.

# Casseroling

Casseroles are a boon to busy people because they can be prepared in bulk, then frozen in suitable portions for those occasions when time is short. You can cut the fat right down when preparing a casserole by:

- Trimming all visible fat away from meat
- Sauteeing onions and garlic in stock or wine
- Chilling the casserole after it's cooked and removing any remaining fat from the surface.

# Grilling

By grilling I mean cooking in a grill pan with heat directly above the food. (Some countries refer to barbecuing as grilling.) Remove grill pan while preheating the grill to high. This prevents food sticking to it when it's placed in the pan.

**Meat**
Place the meat on the grill rack and position the pan as close to the heat as possible. Cook until food is well sealed, about 2–3 minutes, then turn and seal on the other side for the same time. Now, lower the heat and place the grill pan further away from the element; continue cooking until done to taste, turning food from time to time. If meat has been prepared in a marinade which contains honey, jam or a sweet sauce, watch the food carefully, because the sugar in the marinade will attract the heat and the food may scorch easily.

**Fish**
There are certain points to remember when grilling fish. For thick whole fish or thick fillets, it's important to make 2–3 diagonal cuts across the body on both sides—this prevents the fish from curling up and allows for even cooking.

Fillets, cutlets and whole fish should only be turned once while grilling. Brush surface of fish with lemon juice or white wine to prevent it drying out. Cook under moderate heat, allowing 2–3 minutes for thin fillets and 4–5 minutes for thicker pieces, or until flesh flakes when tested with a fork.

# Microwaving

Most households these days have a microwave oven and although I believe they have limitations, there's no denying that they are fast and efficient in cooking vegetables, chicken and fish. And, of course, they reheat food brilliantly. Points to remember are:

- The greater the amount of food to be cooked the longer the cooking time should be.
- Food at room temperature will cook faster than food straight from the refrigerator.
- Microwaving cooks foods from the outside of a dish to the inside, so stir casseroles, soups, etc. once or twice during cooking/reheating.
- Irregularly shaped food, for example fish fillets and chicken breasts, should be placed with the thickest part to the outside of the dish where they will receive more energy.
- Use small pieces of foil to shield areas which attract the most microwave energy, for example chicken wing tips and the corners of square or rectangular dishes.
- Cover food in a microwave if you would normally cover it on a stove or in a conventional oven.
- When cooking fish fillets, allow 1 minute per 100g (3 ounces) on medium high (allow 50 seconds more for thicker fillets) or until flesh flakes.
- Whole fish: small fish require 3–4 minutes on medium power; large fish require 6 minutes per 750g (24 ounces) on medium power.
- When cooking scallops in a browning dish allow 20–30 seconds per 125g (4 ounces) on high heat. Without a browning dish, i.e. cooking in lemon juice, stock or wine, allow 1–2 minutes per 125g (4 ounces) on medium heat.
- Green prawns in a marinade require 2 minutes per 125g (4 ounces).

# Roasting/baking

**Meat**

Preheat oven to required temperature. Trim roast of any fat and weigh to calculate cooking time. Place meat on a rack (or on a bed of julienne vegetables) in a roasting pan. Spray lightly with olive oil. Pour 1 cup of water into base of roasting pan and cook for required time, basting with pan juices from time to time. When cooked, remove from oven, cover loosely with foil and allow to stand for 10–15 minutes before carving. Remove any fat from the pan juices, then deglaze the pan using a little wine or stock combined with the pan juices. Reduce until thickened slightly, or thicken with a little cornflour mixed to a paste with water. Carve roasts across the grain to ensure tenderness.

**Seafood**

Most small or large whole fish, fillets or cutlets can be baked in the oven at 180°C (375°F), unless a recipe specifies another temperature. Whole fish may be stuffed before baking. Place fish into an ovenproof dish or casserole with seasonings and a liquid such as low-fat milk, wine or tomato juice, covered or uncovered, and bake until tender. Fish can also be placed in foil or baking paper and parcelled with other ingredients such as fresh herbs, vegetables and sauces, for aromatic low-fat cooking.

# Steaming

This is an old-fashioned method of cooking but it does produce lovely results with delicate foods such as fish, chicken, eggs, fruit and vegetables. Steamed food loses less of its nutrients than boiled. Simple steamed fish, seafood or chicken can be served Japanese-style with dipping sauces of soy, ginger and wasabi, or try some Thai sweet chilli sauce. You can use:

- Purpose-designed steaming pans.
- Single or multi-layered Chinese bamboo baskets.
- Simple metal steaming baskets which fit inside saucepans (available from kitchen and hardware stores).
- A round cake rack inside a lidded wok.

Whatever equipment you use, there are a few important points to remember when steaming food:

- The food should be protected from the steam by covering lightly with aluminium foil or greaseproof paper.
- The water must be kept boiling throughout the cooking time.
- The saucepan should have a tightly fitting lid so that the steam doesn't escape.
- The steamer must not be allowed to boil dry.
- Allow about one and a half times as long for steaming as boiling.

# Stir-frying

The secret of successful stir-frying is to have all ingredients ready-prepared in bite-size pieces, then cook them quickly over a high heat. Meat diced or cut into strips can be marinated before cooking to add extra flavour and tenderise it.

Heat 2 teaspoons of canola oil in a wok over high heat. Stir-fry meat in small batches for 1–2 minutes, then remove with slotted spoon. Reheat the wok and add the vegetables. Stir-fry for a couple of minutes until they are a vivid colour. Return meat to the wok and add a sauce or the remaining marinade if you like. Stir-fry for 1–2 minutes to heat through, then serve.

---

### Reducing fat in recipes

Most traditional recipes start by frying onions and garlic in oil. If you use a non-stick pan you can reduce that amount to about a teaspoon—that's a saving of 35 grams of fat. You can also soften onion and garlic in stock or wine instead of oil, which adds extra flavour and cuts down the fat even further.

If a recipe calls for initial frying of vegetables, as in moussaka, try spraying them lightly with olive or canola oil, then grilling them instead. They'll cook just as well with a fraction of the fat.

If a favourite recipe involves frying, think of another way to cook it. Marinating meat in a no-oil marinade, then baking it in the oven, results in fantastic flavours. Barbecuing and char-grilling give the same delicious caramelised flavour to meat and chicken as pan-frying, but without the fat. As for fish, it cooks beautifully in its own juices in the microwave.

Make a sauce or gravy from pan juices by draining off the fat, deglazing the pan with stock or wine, then reducing it or thickening with cornflour and water.

Use non-fat yoghurt whenever sour cream is called for and substitute buttermilk for cream in salad dressings. For dishes that require a cheese sauce, try using low-fat ricotta or cottage cheese instead, then sprinkling the top with a little freshly grated Parmesan cheese. The result won't be exactly the same, but the flavour and texture will be just as pleasing.

So don't throw away your cookbooks. Look at your favourite recipes and see how you can adapt them by reducing the fat content. It's really quite easy. You won't compromise the flavour but you'll slash the fat.

# Part II

## Delicious low-fat recipes

# Introduction

Now that you're committed to losing that excess fat through eating well, here are some recipes to get you started. I've tried to use as many different cooking techniques as possible so that you will have practical examples of how you can convert your favourite dishes to low-fat versions.

Longing for a favourite dish often causes resolve to crumble when we're looking for comfort food. However, in most cases high-fat recipes can be converted to low-fat versions without any noticeable loss of flavour. For instance, when the weather is cold and rainy and life isn't at its sparkling best, I always get a hankering for good old spaghetti bolognese or shepherd's pie. Now, these simple, unsophisticated dishes are usually loaded with fat, but I've devised a way to cut the fat right down by sautéing the onions and garlic in stock or wine instead of oil, and using low-fat ingredients. So I can still enjoy all the flavour without worrying that this dish is going to metamorphose into a new spare tyre for my midriff.

Each recipe has an approximate kilojoule (calorie) and fat count per portion size (calculated from the items listed in the ingredients—they do not include serving suggestions). These figures can only be approximate as ingredients can vary with the season, their degree of freshness and place of origin, but they will give you a guide as to how to fit them into your daily fat and energy count.

Most of the recipes are for two people. This is because almost half the households in Australia consist of one or two people and it's easier to halve a recipe for one person, or double it for four, than it is to work out what a single portion would require from a recipe for four or six people. There are instances, however, where larger servings are appropriate, as when you're entertaining, so in that chapter I've made the recipes for four or six people. Where it is not practical to make individual servings (with sauces, for example), I have given recommendations for how long the recipe can be stored.

I hope you enjoy these dishes and that cooking them will encourage you to experiment in the kitchen to create your own low-fat recipes, so that you and your family and friends can enjoy wonderful food and the joy of eating while maintaining a healthy weight and bodily well-being.

# 9  Breakfasts

To successfully lose excess body fat, it is vitally important to eat breakfast as this revs up your metabolism and keeps it burning at a higher level throughout the day. Even if you don't feel very hungry try to have at least one of the nourishing drinks in the chapter.

## Apricot yoghurt smoothie

1 cup unsweetened apricot halves
1 cup non-fat plain yoghurt
1/2 cup skim milk
2 teaspoons honey
3 ice cubes

Place all ingredients in a food processor and blend until smooth.
Serves 2

Per serve: 707kJ/168Cals/0.25g fat

## Mixed berry smoothie

300ml skim milk
1 cup mixed berries (strawberries, raspberries, blackberries, etc.)
1/2 cup fruits of the forest low-fat yoghurt
4 ice cubes

Place all ingredients into a food processor and blend until smooth and frothy. Serve immediately.
Serves 2

Per serve: 361kJ/86Cals/ 0.18g fat

# Mango yoghurt breakfast drink

200g non-fat plain yoghurt
1 cup mango flesh, fresh or canned
1/2 cup skim milk
3 ice cubes

Place all ingredients into a food processor and blend until combined and frothy. Serve immediately.
Serves 2

Per serve: 647kJ/154Cals/0.25g

# Mixed fruit breakfast cocktail

1 cup dried fruit cocktail (apples, apricots, prunes, pears, etc.)
1 cup water
1/2 tablespoon brown sugar
1/2 teaspoon grated fresh ginger
1 tablespoon lemon juice
1/4 teaspoon mixed spice

The night before, place the dried fruit in a bowl. Combine the remaining ingredients in a small pan and heat until just beginning to simmer. Remove from heat, stir well and pour over fruit. Cover and stand overnight. Serve with non-fat yoghurt, if liked.
Serves 2

Per serve: 678kJ/166Cals/0g fat

# Fruit muesli

1/2 cup rolled oats
1 tablespoon sunflower seeds
4 dried apricots, chopped
4 dried dates, chopped
150ml water
1 tablespoon liquid honey
1 large banana
125g seedless green grapes
grated zest 1 orange
grated zest 1 lemon

The night before, place the oats, sunflower seeds, apricots and dates into a bowl. Pour over the water, cover and leave to soak. Next morning, add remaining ingredients. Serve with non-fat plain yoghurt which has been sweetened with a little honey.
Serves 2

Per serve: 1297kJ/308Cals/1.5g fat

# Rice with apple and yoghurt

This is a nutritious breakfast using leftover brown rice.

1 cup cooked brown rice
1 tablespoon wheat germ
1 tablespoon oat bran
1 large Red Delicious apple, grated with skin
1 teaspoon lemon juice
2 tablespoons sultanas
2 tablespoons non-fat plain yoghurt
1 teaspoon honey

Place the rice into a bowl and stir through the wheat germ and oat bran. Combine the grated apple and lemon juice and stir through the rice with the sultanas. Combine the yoghurt and honey. Serve rice and apple mixture with yoghurt.
Serves 2

Per serve: 1293kJ/307Cals/3g fat

---

## Eggs

Eggs are highly nutritious and make the perfect breakfast food once or twice a week.
Chicken eggs, poached or boiled:

large—60g = 375kJ/7g fat
medium—53g = 335kJ/6g fat
small—48g = 290kJ/5.5g fat

Duck eggs:

large, 100g = 1025kJ/12g fat

# Pancakes with yoghurt and berries

The batter will make about 4–6 pancakes. Make up all the mixture, interleave the extra pancakes with greaseproof paper, wrap in plastic wrap and foil and freeze for later use.

1/4 cup plain flour
1 tablespoon caster sugar
1 small egg
1 extra egg white
1/4 cup skim milk
1/2 cup thick-style non-fat yoghurt
1 tablespoon honey
1 small punnet berries (strawberries, raspberries, blueberries or a mixture)
extra caster sugar
1/2 lemon

Sift the flour and sugar into a large bowl. Beat the egg and egg white together until combined. Stir in the milk. Add to flour a little at a time, stirring to achieve a pouring batter (you may have to add a little more milk). Combine the yoghurt and honey. Wash the berries and halve if large.

Heat a small, non-stick frying pan over medium heat. Pour in 1/4 cup of batter. Swirl batter around the pan to cover the bottom. As soon as the base is set flip it over to cook the other side. Remove from pan and keep warm. Make three more pancakes. Spread 1/4 cup yoghurt over each pancake, fill with berries, sprinkle with caster sugar and a squeeze of lemon juice, then fold pancake over berries. Serve immediately.
Serves 2

Per serve: 1028kJ/244Cals/3g fat

# Pancakes with mushrooms, ham and corn

The amount of batter in this recipe will make about 4–6 pancakes. Make up the extra pancakes, interleave with greaseproof paper, wrap in plastic wrap and foil and freeze for later use.

1/4 cup plain flour
pinch salt (optional)
1 small egg
1 extra egg white
1/4 cup skim milk
1 cup creamed corn
60g button mushrooms, sliced
2 thin slices lean leg ham (approx. 50g), trimmed of any fat

Sift the flour and salt into a large bowl. Beat the egg and egg white together until combined. Stir in the milk. Add to flour a little at a time, stirring to achieve a pouring batter (you may have to add a little more milk). Place the creamed corn into a small saucepan with the mushrooms, simmer gently for 4–5 minutes or until mushrooms are just cooked.

Heat a small, non-stick frying pan over medium heat. Pour in 1/4 cup of batter. Swirl batter around the pan to cover the bottom. As soon as the base is set flip it over to cook the other side.

Place a slice of ham on the pancake and spoon over corn and mushrooms. Fold pancake into quarters and serve.
Serves 2

Per serve: 903kJ/215Cals/3g fat

# Corn, ham and mushroom bagels

1 cup creamed corn
50g lean leg ham, chopped
4 button mushrooms, sliced
salt and pepper to taste
2 bagels, cut in half
1 tablespoon chopped parsley

Place the creamed corn in a small saucepan with the ham and mushrooms. Simmer gently until mushrooms are cooked and moisture has evaporated slightly. Season to taste with salt and pepper. Toast the bagels and top each half with corn mixture. Serve sprinkled with parsley.
Serves 2

Per serve: 1125kJ/267Cals/ 4.5g fat


# Cheese and bean muffins

2 English muffins
3/4 cup salt-reduced baked beans
2 tablespoons Parmesan cheese
ground paprika

Split muffins in half and toast lightly. Heat baked beans until warmed through. Preheat grill to medium hot and line grill pan with foil. Place muffin halves on tray and top with beans and sprinkle with cheese and paprika. Grill until just starting to brown. Serve immediately.
Serves 2

Per serve: 1220kJ/290Cals/4.5g fat

# Easy breakfast kedgeree

This is a great way to use up leftovers. It makes a more substantial weekend breakfast or brunch.

1 cup cooked long grain rice
200g smoked cod or haddock, cut into bite-size pieces
2 spring onions, chopped
1/2 small red capsicum, diced
1/4 cup frozen peas
1/4 cup corn kernels
1 teaspoon hot Madras curry powder (or curry powder of choice)
1/4 cup soy sauce (salt-reduced)
1 tablespoon chicken stock
1 tablespoon chopped parsley

Preheat oven to 200°C. Combine the rice, fish, spring onions, capsicum, peas, corn and curry powder. Place into a baking dish and pour over combined soy sauce and chicken stock. Cover dish with foil and cook for 15 minutes. Remove foil, toss rice, and continue cooking for a further 10–15 minutes. Serve sprinkled with chopped parsley.
Serves 2

Per serve: 1037kJ/247Cals/2.25g fat

# Chicken sausages and baked beans

To speed preparation time, use a food processor to mince the ingredients.

1 small onion, finely minced
2 small chicken breasts, minced
1/4 cup fresh white breadcrumbs
1 egg white
1/2 tablespoon finely chopped parsley
1/4 teaspoon ground sage
salt and pepper to taste
1 cup salt-reduced baked beans

Preheat oven to 220°C. Combine all ingredients except beans in a bowl. With wet hands form chicken mixture into sausage shapes and place on squares of foil. Roll up into a cigar shape and twist ends up to seal. Place seam-side up in a baking dish. Bake for 10–15 minutes or until cooked through.

Meanwhile heat beans in a small saucepan. Serve chicken sausages with beans, accompanied with fresh crusty bread or toast, if liked.
Serve 2

Per serve: 1287kJ/306Cals/4g fat

# 10 Lunch dishes

## Pumpkin and apple soup

This soup is quick to prepare, and will keep in the refrigerator for 2–3 days; it also freezes well. Served with crusty wholegrain bread, it makes a delicious lunch.

6 cups chicken stock
1kg butternut pumpkin, chopped
2 Granny Smith apples, peeled and chopped
2 onions, peeled and chopped
2 cloves garlic, crushed
2 stalks celery, chopped
1 teaspoon ground cumin
1/2 teaspoon ground nutmeg
freshly ground black pepper to taste
2 tablespoons non-fat yoghurt
chopped parsley

Place all ingredients in a large saucepan. Bring to the boil, skim the surface of any scum, reduce heat and simmer for 10–15 minutes or until pumpkin is tender. Puree until smooth. Serve soup with a dollop of yoghurt, sprinkled with parsley.
Serves 8

Per serve: 441kJ/105Cals/0g fat

# Corn, potato and broccoli soup

Here's another tasty soup that's packed full of goodness. It will keep in the fridge for 2–3 days and also freezes well. If the broccoli is fresh and young you can use the stem in the soup as well as the florets—just trim away the end and leaves.

4 cups chicken stock
1 large head broccoli (about 500g), cut into florets
2 large potatoes, peeled and chopped
1 onion, peeled and chopped
1 bay leaf
2 stalks parsley
425g can sweet corn kernels
salt, pepper and freshly ground nutmeg to taste

Place the stock, broccoli, potatoes, onion, bay leaf and parsley into a saucepan. Simmer for 15–20 minutes or until the vegetables are tender, skimming off any scum which rises to the surface.

Remove bay leaf and parsley. Puree soup until smooth. Return to pan, stir in the sweet corn and season to taste with salt, pepper and nutmeg. Serve with a dollop of yoghurt, if liked.
Serves 6

Per serve: 648kJ/154Cals/1.7g fat

# Banana and cheese pita pockets

If you use Gold Finger bananas for this dish, they don't go brown when cut, so you can omit the lemon juice.

2 tablespoons cracked wheat
1 small banana, sliced
1/2 tablespoon lemon juice
1/2 large orange, peeled and chopped
2 tablespoons chopped fresh parsley
2 tablespoons sultanas
30g grated Swiss cheese
freshly ground black pepper to taste
2 pita pockets

Soak cracked wheat in cold water for 1 hour. Drain well. Toss banana in lemon juice then combine with remaining ingredients, except pita pockets. Slice open pita pockets, leaving some section of the edge intact. Fill pockets with banana cheese mixture and press openings closed.
Serves 2

Per serve: 1627kJ/387Cals/5.5g fat

# Tuna, corn and lettuce pockets

80g can sandwich tuna in brine
1/2 cup creamed corn
4 cherry tomatoes, sliced
salt and pepper to taste
4 cos lettuce leaves, torn into small pieces
2 pita pockets

In a bowl combine the tuna, corn, tomatoes and salt and pepper. Cut along the edge of the pita pockets halfway round so that they open up. Place lettuce inside the pita pockets. Spoon in the tuna filling and press opening closed.
Serves 2

Per serve: 1086kJ/258Cals/2.3g fat

# Asparagus mornay

1 bunch asparagus spears, trimmed
2 crusty rolls, halved
1 tablespoon Dijon mustard
1/2 cup mornay sauce (see recipe page 200)
ground paprika

Poach, steam or microwave asparagus until tender crisp. Drain and cut in half. Preheat grill to medium hot. Spread rolls with mustard and top with asparagus. Spoon over mornay sauce and sprinkle with paprika. Grill until bubbling and turning golden brown.
Serves 2

Per serve: 936kJ/222Cals/3.5g fat

# Beef and capsicum salad

250g rump steak, trimmed of all fat
freshly ground black pepper
mixed salad greens (include some bitter leaves such as chicory)
1/2 small red capsicum, cut into strips
1 small red onion, sliced into rings
1 small clove garlic, mashed
1½ tablespoons lemon juice
1 tablespoon chopped fresh coriander
1/2 tablespoon fish sauce
1/2 tablespoon brown sugar
basil sprigs for garnish

Sprinkle the steak with pepper and char-grill or sear in a non-stick, ridged frypan until cooked to taste. Remove and allow to stand for 10 minutes.

Meanwhile, place the salad greens, capsicum and onion into a bowl. Combine remaining ingredients and pour over salad. Toss well. Place salad onto serving plates and arranged sliced steak on top. Serve garnished with extra basil leaves.
Serves 2

Per serve: 780kJ/185Cals/3.75g fat

# Prawn and crab salad

This is a great way to use up leftover rice and vegetables. Quick to make, it tastes great.

1½ cups cold cooked rice
125g shelled and deveined prawns
100g crab meat, drained
100g marinated mussels or scallops, drained
2 button mushrooms, sliced
2 tablespoons corn kernels
2 tablespoons cold, cooked peas
1 spring onion, finely chopped
1/4 cup white wine vinegar
1 tablespoon dry sherry
1/2 tablespoon soy sauce
1/2 tablespoon sugar
1/4 teaspoon grated ginger (optional)

Combine rice, seafood and vegetables in a large bowl and toss well. Combine remaining ingredients and pour over salad. Toss well and serve immediately.
Serves 2

Per serve: 1450kJ/345Cals/3.87g fat

---

### In defence of avocado

If you avoid avocado because you think it's 'loaded with fat', you are not only denying yourself a delicious food but one that is extremely good for you. It's true that avocado is high in fat, but it's good-for-our-health fat—monounsaturated fat, the same kind as olive oil. It's an excellent source of folate and vitamin C and a good source of riboflavin, niacin and vitamin A. It also has moderate amounts of iron,

---

# Ham and orange slaw

50g lean leg ham, cut into strips
1 cup shredded green cabbage
1 small red onion, sliced
1 small navel orange, peeled and segmented
1 tablespoon chopped walnuts
1/4 cup fresh orange juice
1/4 tablespoon chopped fresh parsley
1/2 tablespoon apple cider vinegar
1 teaspoon brown sugar

Combine the ham, cabbage, onion, orange and walnuts in a bowl. Combine remaining ingredients, stirring until sugar dissolves. Pour over slaw. Toss to dress well.
Serves 2

Per serve: 479kJ/114Cals/4g fat

---

potassium and thiamine. So eating avocado in moderation is a very healthy food choice, so long as you take its fat and kilojoule content into consideration. For example:

- A slice of avocado that you might have in a sandwich (approx. 10g) has 65kJ/16Cals and 1.5g fat
- 1/2 small avocado has 370kJ/88Cals and 9g fat
- 1 tablespoon of mashed avocado (approx. 20g) has 135kJ/32Cals and 3g fat.

So spread avocado on your sandwich. Butter and margarine have 605kJ/145Cals and 16g fat per tablespoon, and mayonnaise has 565kJ/135Cals and 14g fat per tablespoon, without any of the nutritional benefits of avocado.

# Chicken noodle salad

1/2 cup chopped, cooked chicken breast meat (no skin)
1/2 small green capsicum, diced
1/2 small red capsicum, diced
1 small clove garlic, crushed
1 tablespoon snipped chives
100g dry plain noodles
1 tablespoon soy sauce (salt-reduced)
1/2 tablespoon dry sherry
1/2 teaspoon sesame oil
1/4 teaspoon grated fresh ginger

Place the chicken into a bowl with the capsicum, garlic and chives and mix well.

Cook noodles in plenty of boiling water according to packet directions. Drain. Combine the soy sauce, sherry, sesame oil and ginger. Toss all ingredients together well and serve.
Serves 2

Per serve: 1010kJ/240Cals/2.9g fat

---

### Use your noodle

For a quick tasty lunch, simply simmer some vegetables in stock, then add strips of meat or seafood. Cook for 2–3 minutes, then stir in some 2-minute noodles and cook until tender. Delicious, easy, and very low in fat!

---

# Warm baby octopus salad

300g baby octopus
1/4 cup dry white wine
1 tablespoon sweet chilli sauce
grated zest and juice 1 lime
grated zest and juice 1/2 orange
1 teaspoon brown sugar
1/2 teaspoon fish sauce
1/4 teaspoon grated fresh ginger
mixed salad greens

Wash octopus and pat dry with paper towel. Place in a bowl. Combine the wine, chilli sauce, lime and orange zest and juice, brown sugar, fish sauce and ginger. Pour over octopus, making sure they are well coated. Cover and marinate for at least 1 hour. The longer the marinating time the better the flavour—they can be marinated for up to 24 hours if covered and refrigerated.

Heat a non-stick wok or frypan over medium high heat. Tip both octopus and marinade into the pan and stir-fry quickly for 3–5 minutes or until octopus are just cooked—overcooking will toughen them. Remove from the heat and cool briefly.

Arrange the salad greens in a bowl and pour octopus and pan juices over, toss well and serve.
Serves 2

Per serve: 696kJ/165Cals/1.9g fat

# Salmon burgers
## (*microwave*)

210g pink salmon, drained, skin and bones removed
2 spring onions, very finely chopped
2 tablespoons peeled cucumber, finely chopped
1/3 cup fresh breadcrumbs
1 egg white
1 teaspoon freshly squeezed lemon juice
2 tablespoons wholemeal breadcrumbs for coating
2 teaspoons ground paprika
4 hamburger buns

Combine salmon, spring onions and cucumber in a bowl. With wet hands shape into patties. Dip in combined egg white and lemon juice. Coat in breadcrumbs combined with paprika and place on a microwave-safe plate. Cover with greaseproof paper and microwave on High (100% power) for 3–5 minutes, turning over halfway through. Serve in toasted hamburger buns with sliced tomato, beetroot, lettuce or whatever you like.
Serves 2

Per serve: 1405kJ/335Cals/9.5g fat

# Crab cakes with cucumber relish

210g crab meat, drained
100g boneless white fish fillet
1 large egg white
1/2 teaspoon minced coriander
1/2 teaspoon minced garlic
1/2 teaspoon minced ginger
1/2 teaspoon minced chilli
1 spring onion, sliced
1/2 cup dried wholemeal breadcrumbs
2 tablespoons ground paprika
Cucumber relish:
1/2 cup peeled, seeded cucumber, finely chopped
1 tablespoon sugar
1 tablespoon lemon juice
1/2 teaspoon minced chilli

Place crab, fish fillet, egg white, coriander, garlic, ginger, chilli and spring onion into a food processor. Process until smooth. With wet hands form into 4 flat cakes. Coat with breadcrumbs combined with paprika. Place on a microwave-safe plate and cook on High (100% power) for 3–5 minutes or until cooked. Combine all relish ingredients. Refrigerate until ready to serve. Serve crab cakes with cucumber relish and a green salad.
Serves 2

Per serve: 1151kJ/274Cals/1.75g fat

# Potato with chicken and corn

Quick, tasty, nourishing—what more could you want from a meal?

1 Desiree or other baking potato (about 250g)
1/4 cup creamed corn
1/3 cup chopped cooked chicken
1/4 teaspoon dried coriander (optional)
1 tablespoon chopped fresh parsley

Scrub potato and pierce two or three times with a skewer. Place on a sheet of paper towel in the centre of the turntable of your microwave. Microwave for 4 minutes on High (100% power), turning over halfway through cooking. Remove from oven and wrap in foil. Allow to stand for 5 minutes.

Meanwhile, heat creamed corn, chicken and coriander together in a small saucepan or in the microwave. When potato is ready, place onto warmed serving plate and slit in half. Fill with chicken and corn and serve sprinkled with parsley.
Serves 1

Per serve: 1407kJ/335Cals/3g fat

# Jacket potatoes with beans and ham

This is an extremely simple but highly nutritious lunchtime meal.

1 Desiree or other baking potato (about 250g)
1/2 cup salt-reduced baked beans
30g lean leg ham, chopped
1 tablespoon chopped fresh parsley

Scrub potato and pierce two or three times with a skewer. Place on a sheet of paper towel in the centre of the turntable of your microwave. Microwave for 4 minutes on High (100% power), turning over halfway through cooking. Remove from oven and wrap in foil. Allow to stand for 5 minutes.

Meanwhile, heat beans and ham together in a small saucepan or in the microwave. When potato is ready, place onto warmed serving plate and slit in half. Fill with beans and ham and serve sprinkled with parsley.
Serves 1

Per serve: 1514kJ/360Cals/3.4g fat

# Quick fish lunch

For those occasions when you can have a proper meal at lunch time, here's a very quick microwave dish—it only takes about 12 minutes to prepare and cook. The sauces and juice from the fish make a tasty gravy to add interest to the vegetables.

180g ling fillet
1 tablespoon Thai sweet chilli sauce
1 teaspoon soy sauce (salt-reduced)
1/2 small carrot
1 small zucchini
1 small piece pumpkin, about 2.5cm by 10cm
1 Desiree or other baking potato, about 200g, scrubbed

Place the fish into a microwave-safe dish, spread with Thai chilli sauce and sprinkle with soy sauce. Cover with plastic wrap. Using a potato peeler, cut carrot, zucchini and pumpkin into ribbons. Place in another microwave dish and cover with plastic wrap. Pierce the potato in one or two places and place on microwave turntable. Cook on High (100% power) for 4 minutes, turning over halfway through cooking. Wrap in foil and stand while preparing other ingredients.

Microwave fish on High for 2 minutes. Allow to stand while preparing vegetables. Microwave ribboned vegetables on High for 45 seconds or until tender but still crisp. Place fish onto a serving plate with jacket potatoes and vegetables and spoon fish juices over.
Serves 1

Per serve: 1475kJ/351Cals/2.7g fat

# 11 Beef, lamb, pork and veal

## BEEF

## Beef stock

It's well worth taking the time to make your own stock. Not only does it taste superior to commercial products, but you can control the amount of salt used, making it far healthier for you. Stock can be made, then frozen in 1 cup amounts or in ice cube trays—small portions for sweating vegetables. Once cubes have frozen, unmould them and store in freezer bags. Frozen beef stock will keep for 6–12 months.

3kg beef bones
1 leek (white part only), washed
3 medium carrots, washed
1/2 bunch celery, washed and chopped
2 large onions, peeled and chopped
small bunch parsley
3 cloves
3 bay leaves
salt and pepper to taste

Rinse bones under cold running water, then place in a large saucepan. Cover with water and place over medium heat. Bring to the boil, skimming any scum from the surface. Add remaining ingredients and simmer for at least 4 hours, skimming surface from time to time. Strain, being careful not to let any sediment through. Chill, remove any fat, then use or freeze.
Makes about 3 litres

Per cup: 115kJ/27Cals/0g fat

# Beef, vegetables and noodles

This dish is a cross between a casserole and an Asian-style soup. It's extremely quick to make, satisfying and delicious.

1 small onion, cut into thin wedges
1 clove garlic, crushed
2 cups good beef stock
1/3 small red capsicum, cut into squares
1 cup broccoli florets
1 stalk celery, sliced diagonally
4 spears baby corn, halved
salt and pepper to taste
250g rump steak, sliced into paper-thin strips
100g plain dry noodles

Place the onion and garlic in a saucepan with the beef stock and gently simmer for 2–3 minutes. Add the capsicum, broccoli and celery and continue to simmer for a further 2–3 minutes, or until vegetables are tender but still crisp. Add the corn and warm through. Season to taste.

Cook the noodles according to directions on packet. Just before serving add steak to pan and simmer for just 1 minute, as the meat will cook extremely quickly.

Drain noodles and place in 2 deep soup bowls. Ladle meat and vegetables over, then pour remaining soup on top. Serve immediately.
Serves 2

Per serve: 1613kJ/384Cals/4.87g fat

# Old-fashioned shepherd's pie

Ask your butcher to trim and mince some rump steak for you, or buy steak mince from the supermarket which carries the Heart Foundation Tick of Approval.

1 medium onion, chopped
1 clove garlic, crushed
1¼ cups beef stock
250g lean minced beef
1 carrot, chopped
1 stalk celery, chopped
1 teaspoon Worcestershire sauce
salt and pepper to taste
1 tablespoon cornflour
2 large potatoes, peeled and cut into quarters
ground paprika

Simmer onion, garlic and 1/4 cup stock in a saucepan, stirring occasionally, until onion softens. Increase heat to medium high and add minced beef. Cook, stirring, until it changes colour, breaking up any lumps as it cooks. Reduce heat. Add remaining stock, carrot, celery and Worcestershire sauce, and season to taste with salt and pepper. Cover and simmer gently for 30 minutes or until mince is tender. Mix cornflour to a smooth paste with a little water. Add to pan and stir to combine. Bring to boil, stirring constantly, reduce heat and simmer until thickened.

While mince is cooking, boil potatoes, then mash with skim milk, salt and pepper. Place the mince into a heatproof dish. Top with mashed potatoes. Sprinkle with paprika. Place under a high grill to brown. Serve with peas and corn.
Serves 2

Per serve: 1694kJ/403Cals/8.75g fat

# Stir-fried beef and vegetables

1 tablespoon dry sherry
1 tablespoon soy sauce
1/4 teaspoon grated fresh ginger
1/4 teaspoon chopped fresh chilli
250g rump steak, trimmed and finely sliced
1/4 cup beef stock
1 small onion, petalled
1 small clove garlic, crushed
1 carrot, sliced diagonally
1/2 small red capsicum, cut into bite-sized squares
6 spears baby corn, cut in half
1/2 punnet bean sprouts

Combine the sherry, soy sauce, ginger and chilli in a bowl. Add the beef strips and stir to coat well. Cover and marinate for 30 minutes. Prepare all other ingredients so that they are ready to use.

Heat a non-stick wok or frypan over high heat. Add beef strips and stir-fry quickly until they change colour—this will only take a minute or so. Tip beef strips and any juice they have given off into a bowl.

Reduce heat to medium and return wok to stove. Add the beef stock, onion and garlic and simmer, stirring, until onion has softened. Add remaining ingredients except bean sprouts. Stir-fry vegetables until they become bright in colour and are tender but still crisp.

Return beef and juices to the pan with the remaining marinade and bean sprouts. Toss quickly until meat is heated through. Serve with steamed rice.

Serves 2

Per serve: 999kJ/238Cals/4.37g fat

# Meatballs with tomato sauce

This is a low-fat version of an old-fashioned favourite and is real comfort food, especially on cold winter days. Buy mince with the Heart Foundation Tick of Approval or ask your butcher to trim some rump steak and then mince it for you.

250g minced rump steak
1 spring onion, very finely chopped
1/4 cup fine fresh breadcrumbs
1 tablespoon finely chopped parsley
1/4 teaspoon dried mixed herbs
salt and black pepper to taste
1 egg white
1 onion, chopped
1 clove garlic, crushed
1/4 cup beef stock
2 ripe tomatoes, peeled, seeded and chopped
1/4 cup red wine
$1\frac{1}{2}$ tablespoons tomato paste
2 anchovy fillets, drained on paper towel and mashed
1 tablespoon chopped fresh basil (or 1 teaspoon dried)

In a bowl combine the mince, spring onion, breadcrumbs and herbs. Season to taste with salt and pepper. Mix in the egg white. With damp hands form meat into balls about the size of a walnut. Place on a plate, cover and refrigerate for 15 minutes.

Meanwhile, simmer the onion and garlic in a saucepan with the stock until softened. Add the tomatoes, red wine, tomato paste and anchovies. Simmer gently, stirring occasionally, and breaking up the tomatoes as you do. You may have to adjust the amount of liquid to achieve a simmering sauce, either by adding more stock or evaporating the liquid. Add the meatballs and basil, then simmer gently for 30–40 minutes. Serve with spaghetti, crusty bread and a salad.
Serves 2

Per serve: 1173kJ/279Cals/5.6g fat

# Marinated rump steak

Marinate steak, covered in the refrigerator, in the morning before you head off for the day. Then when you come home all you have to do is grill or barbecue it, toss together some salad greens, open a good bottle of red and you've got a wonderful meal.

300g rump steak, trimmed of all fat
1/4 cup soy sauce (salt-reduced)
1 tablespoon honey
1 tablespoon lemon juice
1 teaspoon ground ginger
1 clove garlic, finely chopped

Place the steak in a shallow dish. Combine remaining ingredients and pour over steak. Cover and marinate for 8 hours. Drain steak, then barbecue or grill until done to taste, brushing with marinade as you turn it. Serve with Microwave Jacket Potatoes (see page 176) and a salad.
Serves 2

Per serve: 960kJ/228Cals/4.5g fat

---

*Here's a dry rub for beef that's great for barbecued steak:* Combine 1 well mashed clove of garlic, 1 teaspoon chilli powder, 1/4 teaspoon dried oregano, 1/4 teaspoon ground cumin and salt and pepper to taste. Rub into meat and allow to stand for at least 30 minutes before cooking.

# Thai beef salad

2 tablespoons lime juice (use lemon if lime is unavailable)
1 tablespoon brown sugar
1 tablespoon fish sauce
1 small clove garlic, crushed
1/2 teaspoon chopped chilli (or to taste)
250g lean beef strips
mixed salad greens of choice

Combine the lime juice, brown sugar, fish sauce, garlic and chilli. Dry-fry beef strips in a non-stick wok or frying pan until cooked to taste. Place salad greens in a serving bowl. Pour lime dressing over and toss well. Pile salad on serving plates and top with beef strips.
Serves 2

Per serve: 857kJ/204Cals/5.5g fat

---

### Beef partners

Low-fat ingredients to combine with beef include: brandy; capsicums; cardamom; celery; chillies; cinnamon; garlic; ginger; green and pink peppercorns; horseradish; leeks; mushrooms; mustard; onions; oyster sauce; paprika; parsley; port; red wine; soy sauce; spinach; tomatoes.

# LAMB

## Mini roast with orange sauce

Mini roasts vary in weight so you may have more than enough for one meal, but leftovers from this dish will make excellent sandwiches the next day.

1 Trim Lamb topside mini roast
1 clove garlic, sliced
1 teaspoon dried rosemary
salt and pepper to taste
1 teaspoon soy sauce (salt-reduced)
1/3 cup orange juice
1 teaspoon grated orange zest

Preheat oven to 180°C. Weigh mini roast to calculate cooking time. With a sharp knife make one or two slits in roast and insert a sliver of garlic in each. Place roast on a rack in a baking dish. Sprinkle with rosemary, salt and pepper. Pour a cup of water into baking dish and bake until done to taste—20–25 minutes per 500g for rare, 25–30 minutes per 500g for medium or 30–35 minutes per 500g for well done.

Remove roast from pan, cover with foil and allow to stand for 10 minutes. Meanwhile, skim fat from juices in baking dish. Pour in the soy sauce, orange juice and zest and stir to deglaze any brown bits sticking to the pan. Pour into a small saucepan and bring to the boil, reduce heat and simmer until reduced and thickened slightly. Serve lamb sliced with sauce spooned over with jacket potatoes and vegetables.
Serves 2

Per serve: 737kJ/175Cals/6.8g fat

# Lamb pilaf

This is a great recipe for using leftover baked lamb—quick, easy and just delicious!

1/4 cup dry white wine
1 small onion, chopped
1 clove garlic, crushed
1 small red capsicum, chopped
1 tomato, peeled and chopped
30g raisins (chopped if large)
1/2 teaspoon ground cinnamon
1/4 teaspoon ground ginger
1/4 teaspoon cardamom seeds
200g cooked lean roast lamb, cut into strips
2 cups cooked long grain rice
freshly ground black pepper
2 tablespoons non-fat skim milk yoghurt
1 tablespoon chopped fresh parsley
1/2 tablespoon grated lemon zest

Place wine in a saucepan and add onion and garlic. Simmer gently, stirring constantly, until onion has softened, about 3 minutes. Add capsicum, tomato, raisins and spices. Stir well and simmer for a further 3 minutes. Add lamb and rice, and season to taste with pepper. Using chopsticks, toss mixture continuously until heated through. Serve with a dollop of yoghurt, and sprinkled with parsley and lemon zest.
Serves 2

Per serve: 1927kJ/458Cals/6g fat

# Lamb and vegetable stew

1 small onion, chopped
1 clove garlic, crushed
1/4 cup dry white wine
250g Trim Lamb, diced
1 carrot, chopped
1 stalk celery, chopped
2 ripe tomatoes, peeled, seeded and chopped
1/4 cup beef stock
1 tablespoon tomato paste
1 teaspoon Worcestershire sauce
salt and freshly ground black pepper to taste

Simmer the onion and garlic in the wine until softened. Add the lamb and remaining ingredients to the saucepan. Cover and cook over very gentle heat for $1\frac{1}{4}$–$1\frac{1}{2}$ hours or until lamb is tender. Serve with jacket potatoes and vegetables of choice.
Serves 2

Per serve: 990kJ/235Cals/6.87g fat

*This simple sauce goes well with grilled lamb:* In a small saucepan combine 2 tablespoons red wine or sherry vinegar, 2 tablespoons redcurrant jelly, 2 tablespoons chopped fresh mint leaves, and salt and pepper to taste. Simmer for 1–2 minutes, stirring well, and serve.

# Lebanese-style lamb meatballs

250g Trim Lamb leg steak, minced
1/2 teaspoon ground cinnamon
1/2 teaspoon ground cardamom
1/4 teaspoon ground nutmeg
100g non-fat plain yoghurt
3/4 cup skim milk
3/4 cup water
1 tablespoon chopped fresh parsley

Combine minced lamb, spices and yoghurt in a bowl. With wet hands, form into meatballs the size of a walnut. Place on a plate, cover and refrigerate for 15 minutes.

Combine the milk and water in a saucepan and bring to a gentle simmer. Add meatballs and poach gently for 8–10 minutes. Sprinkle with parsley. Serve with couscous and side dishes of yoghurt and cucumber, tomato, onion and mint, and banana and sultanas.
Serves 2

Per serve: 1063kJ/253Cals/8.8g fat

# Spicy lamb leg steaks

200g non-fat plain yoghurt
1 tablespoon curry powder
1/2 tablespoon garam masala
2 Trim Lamb topside steaks (about 180g each)
1 tablespoon chopped fresh mint

Combine yoghurt, curry powder and garam masala. Place the lamb steaks in a flat dish and add yoghurt mixture, turning steaks over so that they are coated on both sides. Cover and marinate for 30 minutes.

Drain lamb steaks and grill under medium heat for 2–3 minutes each side or until cooked to taste. Serve lamb sprinkled with mint, and with baby new potatoes and vegetables of choice.
Serves 2

Per serve: 1250kJ/297Cals/8.35g fat

---

### Lamb partners

Low-fat ingredients to combine with lamb include: artichokes; anchovies; capsicum; chickpeas; couscous; eggplants; garlic; grated zest and juice of lemons; mint; mushrooms; onions; parsley; raisins; rosemary; spinach; tomatoes; white wine; zucchini.

---

# Lamb stuffed with apricot and coriander

1 Trim Lamb round mini roast
1 small onion, chopped
1 clove garlic, crushed
1/4 cup dry white wine
1 tablespoon cracked wheat
1/4 cup fresh breadcrumbs
1 tablespoon finely chopped dried apricots
1 tablespoon chopped fresh coriander

Preheat oven to 180°C. Weigh mini roast to calculate cooking time. With a sharp knife, cut a pocket in the side of the mini roast, set aside. Simmer the onion and garlic in the wine in a small saucepan until softened. Add the cracked wheat, breadcrumbs, apricots and coriander. Stuff pocket in mini roast with this mixture. Secure opening with a toothpick or skewer. Place on a rack in a baking dish to which a cup of water has been added.

Roast until done to taste—20–25 minutes per 500g for rare, 25–30 minutes per 500g for medium or 30–35 minutes per 500g for well done. Allow to stand covered in foil for 10 minutes before carving. Serve sliced with a mixed green salad.
Serves 2 (with leftovers)

Per serve: 1126kJ/268Cals/7.5g fat

## Spicy roast pork

1 teaspoon brown sugar
1 teaspoon cracked black pepper
1/2 teaspoon coarse salt
1/2 teaspoon ground coriander
1/2 teaspoon ground cloves
300g pork fillet, trimmed of all fat
1 teaspoon olive oil
1 teaspoon honey

Combine the sugar, pepper, salt, coriander and cloves. Place the pork in a glass dish and rub with the spice mixture, ensuring that it is completely coated. Cover and marinate for 8 hours or overnight.

Preheat oven to 190°C. Place pork on a roasting rack, tucking the thin tail under so that the fillet is an even thickness for all its length. Place rack in a roasting pan and pour in 1 cup of water. Brush meat with olive oil. Roast for 20 minutes. Brush with honey and continue roasting for a further 20 minutes or until pork is cooked, basting with pan juices from time to time. If pan juices are drying out add some more water. Allow to stand for 10 minutes. Strain any fat from pan juices, then place in a saucepan and reduce over high heat until thickened slightly. Serve pork sliced with a coleslaw salad, or with boiled new potatoes and vegetables of choice.
Serves 2

Per serve: 750kJ/178Cals/4g fat

# Soy sherry pork steaks

1 tablespoon soy sauce (salt-reduced)
1 tablespoon medium dry sherry
1 clove garlic, crushed
1/2 teaspoon minced ginger
dash Tabasco sauce
2 pork leg steaks (about 150g each)
1/4 cup chicken stock
1 teaspoon cornflour

Combine the soy sauce, sherry, garlic, ginger and Tabasco sauce. Place steaks in a glass dish and pour marinade over. Cover and allow to marinade for 2 hours. Drain, reserving marinade.

Grill steaks (or cook them on a non-stick, ridged frypan) for about 3–4 minutes or until cooked through.

Meanwhile, place reserved marinade in a small pan and add chicken stock. Mix the cornflour to a paste with a little water and add to the pan. Cook, stirring, until sauce boils and thickens.

Serve pork with baby new potatoes and peas with sauce poured over.
Serves 2

Per serve: 745kJ/177Cals/2.25g fat

*Thai flavoured pork marinade:* Combine 1 tablespoon chopped fresh coriander, 1 tablespoon chopped fresh mint, 1 finely chopped spring onion, 1 chopped small red chilli (or to taste), 1/2 tablespoon fish sauce, 1/2 tablespoon lemon juice, 1 teaspoon brown sugar. Pour over meat and allow to stand for at least 30 minutes before baking, grilling or barbecuing.

# Cider pork kebabs

300g lean diced pork
3/4 cup still cider
2 spring onions, chopped
1 clove garlic, crushed
salt and pepper to taste
1/2 small red capsicum, cut into squares
1/2 small green capsicum, cut into squares
bamboo skewers, soaked in cold water for 30 minutes

Place the pork in a bowl. Combine the cider, onions and garlic and season to taste with salt and pepper. Pour over pork and mix well. Cover and allow to marinate for at least 30 minutes or up to 8 hours (marinate the pork in the morning and it will be ready to cook when you come home after work).

Drain pork and reserve marinade. Thread pork onto skewers alternately with capsicum. Brush with marinade and grill or barbecue until meat is cooked through, about 5 minutes, turning and basting the skewers with the marinade from time to time. Serve with a baked potato and non-fat yoghurt.
Serves 2

Per serve: 795kJ/189Cals/2.25g fat

---

### Pork partners

Low-fat ingredients to combine with pork include: apple; apple brandy; apricots; cabbage; celery; chillies; cider; fennel; garlic; ginger; honey; mushrooms; mustard; onions; pears; prunes; rosemary; sage; soy sauce; thyme; tomatoes; white wine.

---

# Pork chops with redcurrant glaze

1/2 cup red wine
1 teaspoon dried rosemary
2 butterfly steaks (about 300g), trimmed of all fat
2 tablespoons redcurrant jelly
1/2 tablespoon lemon juice
1/2 tablespoon Dijon mustard

Combine the wine and rosemary. Place pork steaks in a flat dish and pour marinade over. Cover and marinate for 30 minutes. Drain well, reserving marinade.

Strain marinade into a small saucepan, add remaining ingredients and stir well to combine. Bring to the boil, reduce heat and simmer until thickened slightly.

Brush pork steaks with redcurrant glaze, then grill until cooked through, approximately 4–5 minutes, brushing with glaze as you turn them. Serve with remaining glaze poured over with yellow squash, carrots and baby new potatoes.
Serves 2

Per serve: 1107kJ/263Cals/2.25g fat

---

*Here's a delicious glaze to use with lamb or pork:* Puree 4 large apricot halves and combine with 1 tablespoon Worcestershire sauce, 1 tablespoon light soy sauce, 1/2 tablespoon brown sugar, 1/2 tablespoon tomato paste, 1 teaspoon grated fresh ginger, dash Tabasco sauce, 1 crushed clove garlic, and pepper to taste. Brush over meat while baking, grilling or barbecuing.

# Apricot pork kebabs

1 clove garlic, crushed
1 tablespoon chilli sauce
1 tablespoon apricot jam
1 teaspoon hoi sin sauce
1 teaspoon cider vinegar
1/2 teaspoon soy sauce (salt-reduced)
300g pork leg steaks
8 dried apricots

Place the garlic, chilli sauce, apricot jam, hoi sin sauce, vinegar and soy sauce in a small saucepan and heat gently, stirring, until combined. Cool.

Cut pork leg steaks into bite-sized pieces. Thread pork and apricots onto wooden skewers, place in a shallow dish and pour chilli apricot marinade over. Turn kebabs in marinade so they are well coated. Cover and marinate for 1 hour or place in the refrigerator and leave to marinate for 8–24 hours. This means you can prepare the recipe the night before or in the morning and have the kebabs ready to cook as soon as you get home from work.

Drain kebabs and reserve marinade. Grill or barbecue kebabs for 8–10 minutes or until cooked through, turning and basting with marinade as they cook. Serve with steamed rice and a salad.
Serves 2

Per serve: 1037kJ/247Cals/2.25g fat

# Baked pork fillet with tomato sherry glaze

300g pork fillet, trimmed of any fat
2 tablespoons dry sherry
1 tablespoon honey
1 tablespoon tomato sauce
1/8 teaspoon five spice powder
1/2 tablespoon soy sauce (salt-reduced)
1/3 cup chicken stock
1 teaspoon oyster sauce
1 teaspoon cornflour

Place pork in a bowl. Combine sherry, honey, tomato sauce, five spice powder and soy sauce. Pour over fillet, coating well. Cover and marinate for 1 hour. Drain, reserving marinade.

Preheat oven to 180°C. Place pork fillet on a rack in a baking dish, tucking the tail under so that it is of an even thickness for all its length. Add half a cup of water to the baking dish. Bake for 20–30 minutes, or until pork is cooked, basting with marinade from time to time.

Place remaining marinade into a small saucepan with the chicken stock and oyster sauce. Bring to the boil, reduce heat and simmer until reduced slightly. Mix cornflour to a paste with a little water. Remove pan from heat and stir in cornflour paste, stirring constantly until combined. Return to heat and cook until sauce boils and thickens. Serve pork sliced with sauce spooned over with baby new potatoes and steamed vegetables.
Serves 2

Per serve: 1060kJ/252Cals/1.5g fat

# VEAL

## Italian-style veal casserole

300g diced veal, trimmed of any fat
1 tablespoon flour seasoned with salt and pepper
2 tomatoes, peeled, seeded and chopped
1 carrot, chopped
1 stalk celery, chopped
1 small onion, chopped
1 clove garlic, crushed
1 small strip orange rind (about 5cm long)
1 bay leaf
1 sprig thyme
1/3 cup dry white wine
1/3 cup chicken stock
1 tablespoon tomato paste
1 tablespoon chopped parsley

Preheat oven to 160°C. Place seasoned flour in a paper bag. Add veal and shake well to coat meat in flour. You may have to do this in batches. Place in a casserole with tomatoes, carrot, celery, onion, garlic, orange rind, bay leaf and thyme.

Combine wine, chicken stock and tomato paste. Pour over meat and vegetables. Cover and bake for about 1–1½ hours or until meat is tender. Remove bay leaf and orange peel. Sprinkle with parsley and serve with spiral pasta and a salad.
Serves 2

Per serve: 1145kJ/272Cals/3.87g fat

# Grilled veal steaks with wine-rosemary baste

1/4 cup dry white wine
1 tablespoon lemon juice
1 clove garlic, crushed
2–3 sprigs fresh rosemary
1 tablespoon chopped fresh parsley
salt and pepper to taste
2 veal steaks (about 180g each)

Combine the wine, lemon juice, garlic, rosemary, parsley and salt and pepper in a bowl. Place veal in a flat dish and pour wine mixture over, turning steaks so they are well coated. Cover and marinate for 30 minutes.

Preheat grill to medium high. Drain veal and cook for 2–3 minutes each side or until cooked through. Meanwhile place marinade in a small pan and simmer until it reduces slightly. Strain. Serve veal with sauce spooned over accompanied by boiled potatoes, grilled eggplant and tomatoes.
Serves 2

Per serve: 873kJ/207Cals/2.7g fat

---

## Veal partners

Low-fat ingredients to combine with veal include: anchovies; artichokes; eggplants; garlic; leeks; grated zest and juice of lemon; marsala; mushrooms; mustard; onions; parsley; rosemary; sage; spinach; tomatoes; white wine.

# Veal and artichoke casserole

300g diced veal, trimmed of any fat
2 large canned artichokes, cut into quarters
2 spring onions, chopped
1 clove garlic, crushed
1¼ cups white wine
2 ripe tomatoes, peeled, seeded and chopped
1 tablespoon tomato paste
2 anchovy fillets, drained on paper towel and mashed
pinch dried mixed herbs

Preheat oven to 180°C. Place the diced veal in a casserole. Arrange artichoke quarters in and around the meat.

Simmer the spring onions and garlic in 1/4 cup of wine until softened, then add the remaining ingredients. Bring to the boil, reduce heat and simmer for 2–3 minutes. Pour over veal in casserole. Cover and bake for 1 hour or until veal is cooked and tender. Serve with spiral pasta and salad.
Serves 2

Per serve: 1397kJ/333Cals/4.7g fat

# Veal marsala

2 large veal schnitzels
canola or olive oil spray
1 clove garlic, crushed
2 spring onions, chopped
1/4 cup white wine
1 tablespoon marsala
60g button mushrooms, sliced
1/2 tablespoon lemon juice
1 tablespoon finely chopped fresh parsley

Spray a non-stick frypan with canola or olive oil and place over medium heat. Quick-cook schnitzels for 1–2 minutes each side, depending on thickness, or until cooked through. Remove and keep warm.

Add the garlic, spring onions and wine to the pan and cook, stirring, until softened and wine has reduced by half. Add the marsala, mushrooms, lemon juice and parsley and continue cooking until mushrooms have softened. Return veal to pan to coat and warm through. Serve veal with sauce spooned over with mashed potatoes and peas.

Serves 2

Per serve: 1107kJ/263Cals/4.5g fat

---

*Try this simple rub for veal:* Combine 1 teaspoon each dried oregano, basil and thyme with grated zest and juice of half a small lemon. Season to taste with salt and pepper. Rub into veal and allow to stand for at least 30 minutes before grilling or barbecuing.

# 12 Poultry

## Chicken stock

I simply can't throw out chicken bones without making stock from them first. It's so easy and the stock so delicious, that I feel it's a waste not to make it. This stock will freeze for 6–12 months and is wonderful for making quick soups, sauces and mouth-watering risottos.

1kg chicken carcass
3 litres water
200ml white wine
salt to taste
1 tablespoon crushed white peppercorns
1 small leek
1 small carrot
2 stalks celery
1 onion, stuck with 2 cloves
1 bay leaf
a few basil stalks

Place the carcass in a large saucepan. Add remaining ingredients and place pan over medium heat. Simmer for 2 hours, skimming the surface from time to time. Strain, being careful not to let any sediment through.
Makes about 6 cups

Per cup: 115kJ/27Cals/0g fat

# Chicken in a pot

This is a cross between a soup and a casserole. Have all the ingredients prepared before you start cooking. Serve the chicken and vegetables in large soup bowls accompanied by crusty French bread.

2 pieces chicken Maryland, skin removed
1 litre chicken stock
2 sprigs fresh thyme
1 bay leaf
salt and pepper to taste
4 baby carrots, scrubbed
1 small leek, white part only, cut into thick rings
1 large potato, peeled and cut into large chunks
1 small parsnip, cut into large chunks
chopped fresh parsley

Place the chicken pieces in a deep-sided, non-stick frypan or casserole. Pour chicken stock over. Add the thyme and bay leaf and season to taste with salt and pepper. Bring gently to simmering point over low heat. Cover and poach chicken for 10 minutes. It's important that the stock is only at a gently rolling simmer, because if it simmers too hard the chicken will become tough.

Place prepared vegetables into pan around chicken and cook for a further 15 minutes or until chicken is tender and cooked through. Remove chicken from the pan and keep warm, covered.

Continue to simmer vegetables for another 5 minutes until cooked through. Place chicken in serving bowl and ladle over vegetables and soup. Serve sprinkled with chopped fresh parsley.
Serves 2

Per serve: 1520kJ/362Cals/4.5g fat

# Spicy chicken parcels

2 tablespoons chicken stock
1½ tablespoons soy sauce (salt-reduced)
1 clove garlic, crushed
1/2 teaspoon five-spice powder
1/4 teaspoon sugar
300g chicken breast, trimmed of skin and fat

Combine all ingredients except chicken in a small bowl. Place each chicken breast on a square of foil large enough to form a parcel. Fold edges of foil up. Sprinkle over combined sauce ingredients. Carefully fold foil round chicken to make a secure parcel. Allow to stand for 30 minutes.

Preheat oven to 180°C. Bake parcels in a shallow dish for 20–30 minutes or until chicken is cooked. Place parcels on warm serving plates to be opened at the table. Serve with steamed rice and vegetables.
Serves 2

Per serve: 745kJ/177Cals/4.5g fat

---

### Poultry partners

Low-fat ingredients that go well with poultry: anchovies; capers; chilli; coriander; cumin; garlic; fennel; hoi sin sauce; zest and juice of lemons; lemon grass; zest and juice of limes; marsala; mushrooms; mustard; non-fat yoghurt; onions, zest and juice of oranges; paprika; parsley; rosemary; soy sauce; tarragon; thyme; tomatoes; white wine.

## Cajun chicken

300g breast fillets, trimmed
1/2 tablespoon dark brown sugar
1/2 tablespoon lime juice
1/2 teaspoon cracked black pepper
1/2 teaspoon chopped red chilli (or to taste)
pinch cayenne pepper
2 spring onions, finely chopped
2 tablespoons non-fat skim milk yoghurt

Place chicken fillets on a plate. Combine the sugar, lime juice, black pepper, chilli and cayenne. Coat chicken with this mixture, cover and refrigerate 30 minutes. Drain, reserving marinade. Char-grill chicken or cook in a ridged frypan for 4–5 minutes each side, or until cooked through, brushing with marinade mixture with each turn. Serve sprinkled with spring onions and a dollop of yoghurt.
Serves 2

Per serve: 827kJ/196Cals/3.75g fat

## Italian chicken

300g chicken breast fillets, cut into bite-sized pieces
1/4 cup chicken stock or dry white wine
2 ripe tomatoes, peeled, seeded and chopped
6 anchovy fillets, drained on paper towel
2 tablespoons chopped black olives
1/2 teaspoon chicken stock powder
1 teaspoon dried Italian herbs

Preheat oven to 180°C. Place chicken in a casserole dish. Combine remaining ingredients and pour over chicken. Cover and bake for 30 minutes, or until cooked. Serve with pasta and a green salad.
Serves 2

Per serve: 1147kJ/273Cals/9.25g fat

# Barbecued tipsy chicken

You can marinate the chicken for up to 24 hours if it's more convenient—prepare the recipe one evening and cook it the next!

2 chicken breast fillets
1½ tablespoons lemon juice
1 tablespoon brandy
1 tablespoon dark marmalade

Marinate chicken in lemon juice, brandy and marmalade for 30 minutes. Drain, then barbecue, grill or cook in a ridged frypan for 4–5 minutes each side until cooked through, brushing with marinade as they cook. Watch fillets carefully because the sugar in the marmalade attracts the heat and they may burn easily.
Serves 2

Per serve: 921kJ/219Cals/3.75g fat


# Barbecued chicken with lemon and paprika

juice 1/2 lemon
2 tablespoons no-oil vinaigrette dressing
1 teaspoon Worcestershire sauce
1/2 teaspoon Dijon mustard
1 teaspoon lemon pepper
300g chicken breast fillets, skin and fat removed
1/2 tablespoon mild paprika

Combine lemon juice, vinaigrette, Worcestershire sauce, mustard and lemon pepper. Brush chicken with lemon mixture, then sprinkle liberally with paprika. Barbecue or grill chicken until cooked through, brushing with any leftover lemon mixture as it cooks. Serve with salad and crusty bread.
Serves 2

Per serve: 800kJ/190Cals/4.5g fat

# Thai chicken salad

2 small chicken breast fillets, cut into bite-sized pieces
1 Lebanese cucumber, chopped
1 small red onion, cut into rings
100g green pawpaw (optional), cut into long thin shreds
1/2 small yellow capsicum, cut into fine shreds
1 tablespoon chopped fresh mint
1 tablespoon white vinegar
1 tablespoon lime juice
1/2 tablespoon fish sauce
1 teaspoon brown sugar
pepper to taste
whole mint leaves for garnish

Heat a non-stick wok or frypan and dry-fry chicken (without added oil), stirring constantly until cooked, about 3 minutes.

Place the cucumber, onion, pawpaw and capsicum in a salad bowl. Combine remaining ingredients. Pour over salad and toss well. Arrange salad on serving plates with chicken on top. Serve garnished with mint leaves.
Serves 2

Per serve: 908kJ/216Cals/4.35g fat

# Lemon grass chicken

2 tablespoons soy sauce
1 tablespoon fish sauce
2 spring onions, chopped
1 stalk lemon grass, finely chopped
1 clove garlic, crushed
1 teaspoon minced ginger
1 teaspoon chopped chilli
grated rind and juice 1 lime
300g chicken breast fillets, cut into bite-sized pieces
100g noodles, cooked

Combine the sauces, onions, lemon grass, garlic, ginger, chilli and lime juice and rind. Place the chicken in a bowl and pour lemon grass mixture over. Stir well to ensure chicken is evenly coated. Cover and marinate for 30 minutes.

Drain chicken, reserving marinade. Stir-fry chicken in a non-stick wok or frying pan for about 3–5 minutes. Pour in reserved marinade and continue cooking until chicken is tender. Serve over hot noodles.
Serves 2

Per serve: 1634kJ/389Cals/5.45g fat

# Chicken tikka

1 tablespoon ground coriander
1 tablespoon ground cumin
1 teaspoon turmeric
1/2 teaspoon ground chilli powder
1 teaspoon grated fresh ginger
2 cloves garlic, crushed
300ml non-fat yoghurt
300g chicken breast fillets, skin and fat removed

Combine all ingredients except chicken. Place chicken into a shallow baking dish and spread yoghurt mixture over, making sure all chicken is well coated. Cover and marinate in the refrigerator for 8–24 hours.

Preheat oven to 180°C. Bake chicken in baking dish with yoghurt for 25–30 minutes or until chicken is cooked. Serve with steamed rice and a green salad.
Serves 2

Per serve: 1100kJ/261Cals/4.87g fat

---

### Marinades for chicken

Marinate skinless chicken pieces or chicken breast fillets in the following then grill or barbecue meat, basting with marinade as it cooks: 1/2 cup unsweetened pineapple juice; 1/4 cup dry white wine; 1 teaspoon chopped fresh ginger; 1 tablespoon grain mustard; 1/2 tablespoon light soy sauce; 1 chopped spring onion.

# Chicken poached in orange sauce

300g chicken breast fillets
1/4 cup sweet white wine
1/4 cup freshly squeezed orange juice
$1\frac{1}{2}$ tablespoons apple juice
1 tablespoon lemon juice
1 tablespoon honey

Trim the chicken fillets of all fat and cut into bite-sized pieces. Place remaining ingredients in a saucepan. Bring to the boil, reduce heat and simmer for 2–3 minutes. Add chicken and continue to simmer gently, stirring occasionally, for a further 5–10 minutes or until cooked through. Serve with rice and a mixed salad which includes some bitter leaves such as chicory, radicchio or Belgian endive.
Serves 2

Per serve: 1007kJ/239Cals/4.5g fat

# Chicken with mustard and tarragon

2 pieces chicken Maryland, skin and fat removed
1 tablespoon Dijon mustard
1 clove garlic, crushed
1 tablespoon lemon juice
$1\frac{1}{2}$ teaspoon dried tarragon
salt and pepper to taste

Preheat oven to 180°C. Place the chicken in a baking dish and coat with combined remaining ingredients. Cover and bake for 30 minutes or until chicken is cooked through. Serve with fresh asparagus and mushrooms.
Serves 2

Per serve: 825kJ/196Cals/4.5g fat

# Chicken with teriyaki glaze

1½ tablespoons soy sauce
1½ tablespoons Worcestershire sauce
1 tablespoon red wine vinegar
1/3 cup dry sherry
1 tablespoon brown sugar
1 clove garlic, crushed
300g chicken breast fillets, trimmed of all fat

Place all ingredients, except chicken, in a small saucepan. Heat gently until combined. Preheat grill and line tray with foil. Place chicken on foil and brush with teriyaki glaze. Grill for 2–3 minutes, brushing with glaze from time to time. Turn chicken over and continue cooking until cooked through, again brushing with glaze. Serve with any remaining glaze spooned over with baby new potatoes and steamed vegetables.
Serves 2

Per serve: 1033kJ/246Cals/4.5g fat

# Tandoori chicken

1/2 cup non-fat plain yoghurt
1 clove garlic, crushed
1 teaspoon curry powder
1/2 teaspoon grated fresh ginger
1/2 teaspoon chopped fresh chilli
1/2 teaspoon chopped fresh mint
salt and pepper to taste
300g chicken breast fillets, skin and fat removed

Combine all ingredients except the chicken. Place chicken in a baking dish and spoon yoghurt mixture over, making sure that the chicken is well coated. Cover and marinate for 8–24 hours in the refrigerator.

Preheat oven to 180°C. Bake chicken in same dish with yoghurt marinade for 25–30 minutes or until chicken is cooked. Serve with boiled rice, microwaved pappadums (see page 185), and side dishes such as cucumber and yoghurt, sliced banana and mango chutney. Serves 2

Per serve: 852kJ/202Cals/4.65g fat

# Chicken with walnuts and apricot sauce

300g chicken breast fillets, trimmed of skin and fat
1 tablespoon chopped walnuts
1/2 cup apricot nectar
2 spring onions, chopped
1 teaspoon Dijon mustard
1 clove garlic, crushed

Preheat oven to 180°C. Arrange chicken fillets in a baking dish. Sprinkle with walnuts. Combine apricot nectar with the spring onions, mustard and garlic and pour over chicken. Bake chicken for 20–30 minutes or until chicken is cooked through. Serve with salad and crusty bread.
Serves 2

Per serve: 980kJ/233Cals/6.5g fat

---

### Dry-rub marinades

*Try this spicy dry marinade for chicken:* Combine 1 tablespoon finely snipped chives, 1 teaspoon ground allspice, 1/2 teaspoon sugar, 1/4 teaspoon ground cinnamon, 1/4 teaspoon dried thyme, dash Tabasco sauce, salt and pepper to taste. Rub into chicken flesh, cover and allow to marinate for at least 30 minutes before baking, grilling or barbecuing.

*Give chicken a Moroccan flavour with this dry rub:* Combine 1 well mashed clove of garlic with 1 teaspoon ground cinnamon, 1/4 teaspoon ground coriander, 1/4 teaspoon ground cumin, 1/4 teaspoon ground ginger and a good pinch ground nutmeg. Rub into meat and allow to stand for at least 30 minutes before cooking.

*This is very simple but tastes great:* Combine 1 well mashed clove of garlic, 1/2 teaspoon dried rosemary and 1 teaspoon grated lemon zest, rub into chicken and stand for at least 30 minutes before cooking.

# Chicken with walnut crust

15g walnuts, very finely chopped
1 tablespoon dried breadcrumbs
1/2 tablespoon grated orange rind
pinch salt (optional)
2 pieces chicken Maryland, skin and fat removed
1 tablespoon melted honey
1 tablespoon redcurrant jelly
1 tablespoon orange juice
1 tablespoon port
1/2 tablespoon sugar

Preheat oven to 180°C. Combine the walnuts, breadcrumbs, orange rind and salt on a plate. Brush chicken with honey and coat in walnut/crumb mixture. Place on a rack in a baking dish and bake for 20–30 minutes or until chicken is cooked.

Meanwhile, combine the redcurrant jelly, orange juice, port and sugar in a small pan and simmer until sauce boils and thickens slightly. Serve chicken with redcurrant sauce poured over with baby new potatoes and vegetables of choice.
Serves 2

Per serve: 1462kJ/348Cals/8.65g fat

*Garlic lemon marinade for chicken:* Combine grated zest and juice of 1 lemon with 1 tablespoon Dijon mustard, 1 well mashed clove of garlic, 1 teaspoon dried mixed herbs and 1 tablespoon white wine. Pour over chicken and allow to marinate for at least 30 minutes.

# Chicken with curry mango glaze

300g chicken breast or thigh fillets, trimmed of skin and fat
1/4 cup mango chutney
1/2 teaspoon curry powder
$1\frac{1}{2}$ tablespoons soy sauce (salt-reduced)
1/2 teaspoon French mustard

Preheat oven to 180°C. Place the chicken in a shallow baking dish. Combine remaining ingredients and pour over chicken, making sure the chicken is well coated. Bake for 20–30 minutes or until chicken is cooked through. Serve with couscous and a green salad.
Serves 2

Per serve: 1025kJ/244Cals/4.5g fat

# Spatchcocks with garlic and coriander

2 spatchcocks, skin removed, washed and dried
1½ tablespoons fish sauce
2 cloves garlic, crushed
2 tablespoons chopped fresh coriander
salt and freshly ground black pepper

Place spatchcocks in a baking dish. Combine remaining ingredients. Pour over spatchcocks. Cover and refrigerate for 2–3 hours.

Preheat oven to 180°C. Bake spatchcocks for 30–40 minutes or until cooked through, basting with juices from time to time. Serve hot or cold with salad.
Serves 2

Per serve: 1108kJ/263Cals/10.8g fat


# Chicken with plum-soy glaze

300g chicken breast fillets, skin and fat removed
1 tablespoon plum sauce
1/2 tablespoon soy sauce
1/2 tablespoon brown sugar
1/2 tablespoon vinegar
1 clove garlic, crushed
1/2 tablespoon hoi sin sauce
1/2 tablespoon tomato sauce

Place the chicken in a shallow baking dish. Combine the remaining ingredients and pour over chicken. Cover and allow to marinate for 1–8 hours. Drain chicken and barbecue or grill until cooked through, brushing with marinade as it cooks. Serve with a salad.
Serves 2

Per serve: 867kJ/206Cals/4.5g fat

# Steamed tarragon chicken with vegetables

juice 1/2 lemon
1 teaspoon dried tarragon
1 tablespoon dry white wine
salt and freshly ground pepper to taste
300g chicken breast fillets, cut into thick strips about 2cm wide
1/2 small red capsicum, cut into squares
1 stalk celery, sliced diagonally
125g button mushrooms, sliced
extra lemon slices

Combine the lemon juice, tarragon and wine. Season to taste. Add chicken strips and stir well to coat. Cover and marinate for 1 hour.

Arrange chicken and vegetables in a steaming basket and steam for 5 minutes over boiling water. Add mushrooms and gently steam for a further 4 minutes. Serve garnished with lemon slices and steamed rice.
Serves 2

Per serve: 825kJ/196Cals/4.5g fat

# 13 Seafood

Succulent seafood—it doesn't just taste great but also does wonders for our health. It's ideal for people on a low-fat diet because it has extremely low levels of fat—lower than most cuts of chicken and much lower than red meat. All seafoods are excellent sources of top quality protein, many important vitamins (especially the B group), and minerals including iodine, zinc, potassium and phosphorus.

## Fish stock

It takes just 25 minutes to make a good fish stock and the difference between using homemade fish stock and the bought product is like chalk and cheese. It can be made into delicious, low-fat sauces to go with grilled or baked fish, and makes wonderfully fragrant soups and casseroles. It can be frozen for 6–12 months.

1kg fish bones (heads, tails, etc.), washed in cold water
1 small leek (white part only), washed and roughly chopped
1 small carrot, roughly chopped
2 stalks celery, chopped
1 onion, stuck with two cloves
1 bay leaf
1 tablespoon chopped fresh dill (or 2 teaspoons dried)

Place bones in a large saucepan with remaining ingredients. Add water to just cover and bring to the boil. As soon as it boils, reduce heat to just simmering. Simmer for just 20 minutes, skimming the surface from time to time. Don't simmer this stock for longer as the stock can become bitter. Strain carefully.
Makes about 2 litres

Per cup: 110kJ/26Cals/0g fat

# Ling in lettuce parcels

You can use a variety of leaves to make fish parcels, such as spinach, cabbage and vine leaves. Using the basic technique of this recipe you can be really inventive using different fish fillets, vegetables and spices—whatever takes your fancy. This dish is also great for entertaining as it's quick to cook and the parcels can be prepared ahead, then refrigerated until required.

1/2 tablespoon teriyaki sauce
1/2 tablespoon honey
grated zest and juice 1/2 orange
pinch chilli powder
1/4 teaspoon minced ginger
300g ling fillets, cut into bite-size pieces
2 large lettuce leaves, thick central vein removed
1 medium carrot, cut into matchsticks
1/2 stalk celery, cut into matchsticks
1 spring onion, cut into 1cm (1/2") pieces
1 cup chicken stock

Combine the teriyaki sauce, honey, orange zest and juice, chilli powder and ginger in a small bowl. Place the fish in a bowl and pour marinade over. Stir to coat well. Cover and marinate for at least 30 minutes.

Place lettuce leaves on a flat plate (you may need to do this individually depending on the size of your microwave), cover and cook on High for 30 seconds, until just wilted. Cool.

Place the vegetables and stock in a bowl, cover and microwave on High for 3–4 minutes until vegetables are tender.

Place lettuce leaves vein-side up on a chopping board and divide fish between each. Fold leaf to enclose fish completely and place seam-side down in a baking dish. Ladle vegetables and stock over. Cover and cook on High for 2–3 minutes, then allow to stand for

2 minutes. Serve fish parcels with vegetables and broth in warmed, deep soup bowls with plenty of crusty multigrain bread to mop up the broth.

Serves 2

Per serve: 811kJ/193Cals/2.25g fat

---

## What to look for when buying fish

*Whole fish*

- lustrous, bright colour
- bright, bulging eyes
- bright gills
- firm flesh which springs back when touched
- pleasant sea smell

*Fillets/cutlets*

- flesh shiny and firm
- doesn't ooze water when touched
- no discolouration
- good shape
- pleasant sea smell

*Shellfish*

- good lustrous colour
- no discolouration, particularly at joints
- shells tightly closed
- pleasant sea smell

## How much to buy

Per person:

- whole fish: 275–350g; head removed and cleaned: 225–275g
- fish fillets and fish portions: 100–175g
- fish cutlets: 175–225g

# Honey prawns

2 tablespoons honey
2 tablespoons dry sherry
1/2 tablespoon soy sauce
1/4 teaspoon minced ginger
1/4 cup fish or chicken stock
1 clove garlic, crushed
2 spring onions, chopped
1 stalk celery, sliced diagonally
60g mushrooms, sliced
6 snow peas, topped and tailed
1/4 cup bamboo shoots
1/4 cup water chestnuts
500g green prawns, peeled, deveined, tails intact

Combine honey, sherry, soy sauce and ginger and set aside. Place the stock, garlic, onions and celery into a wok and cook, tossing with a chopstick as when stir-frying, until onions have softened. Add remaining vegetables and prawns and toss over high heat until prawns just turn opaque. Add honey mixture and toss quickly to coat prawns and heat through. Serve immediately with steamed rice. Serves 2

Per serve: 972kJ/231Cals/1.25g fat

# Spicy Indian seafood

1/2 teaspoon ground cardamom
1/2 teaspoon ground coriander
1/4 teaspoon ground cloves
1/4 teaspoon garam masala
1/4 teaspoon ground fennel seed
1 cup fish or chicken stock
1 small onion
1 clove garlic, crushed
1 teaspoon chopped fresh chilli (or to taste)
1/4 teaspoon grated fresh ginger
1 tablespoon tomato paste
250g green prawns, shelled and deveined
1 calamari hood, cut into bite-sized pieces and scored in a
diamond pattern
125g mussel meat

In a heavy-based non-stick frypan, dry-roast the cardamom, coriander, cloves, garam masala and fennel seed until aromatic, stirring
all the time so that the spices do not burn. Slowly stir in 1/2 cup
of stock, then the onion, garlic, chilli and ginger. Simmer gently
until onion has softened. Stir in the tomato paste, then add the
seafood and cook for 3–4 minutes or until the prawns just turn
opaque. Serve with steamed rice, microwaved pappadums (see page
185), cucumber and non-fat yoghurt, and sliced banana.
Serves 2

Per serve: 1080kJ/257Cals/4.25g fat

# Sweet and sour fish parcels

You will need aluminium foil or baking parchment for this recipe. Serve the unopened parcels on a dinner plate and open them just before eating. The aroma is delightful. Serve with microwaved or steamed vegetables such as chat potatoes, yellow squash and broccoli.

300g barramundi fillets (2 pieces)
salt and pepper to taste
1/2 tablespoon tomato sauce
1/2 tablespoon soy sauce
1/2 tablespoon honey
1/2 tablespoon dry sherry
1/2 tablespoon orange juice
pinch cayenne pepper

Preheat oven to 180°C. Tear off two pieces of foil large enough to enclose each fish fillet in a parcel. Place fish on foil and season to taste with salt and pepper. Pull the edges up around fish so that the sauce will not run out.

Combine remaining ingredients and pour over fish. Fold foil around fish into a secure parcel. Bake in the oven for 20 minutes until flesh flakes easily with a fork.
Serves 2

Per serve: 559kJ/133Cals/2g fat

# Ling and vegetable casserole

2 zucchinis, cut into julienne strips
1 tomato, peeled and chopped
1 small carrot, cut into julienne strips
1 small onion, sliced
60g mushrooms, sliced
300g ling, cut in cubes
salt and freshly ground pepper to taste
1 cup tomato juice
1 teaspoon Worcestershire sauce
dash Tabasco sauce

Preheat oven to 180°C. Place vegetables in an ovenproof dish. Place fish on top of the vegetables and season to taste with salt and pepper. Pour over combined tomato juice, Worcestershire and Tabasco sauces. Bake for 25 minutes, or until fish flakes easily with a fork. Serve with crusty bread to mop up the juices and a green salad.
Serves 2

Per serve: 757kJ/180Cals/2g fat

# Snapper and vegetable bake

300g snapper fillets, cut into bite-size pieces
1 small red capsicum, diced
1/2 cup corn kernels
2 spring onions, finely chopped
2 teaspoons plain flour
salt and freshly ground black pepper to taste
1 cup low-fat cottage cheese
1/4 cup dried breadcrumbs
1 tablespoon finely chopped parsley
1 tablespoon Parmesan cheese

Preheat oven to 180°C. Combine the fish, capsicum, corn, spring onions and flour in a bowl. Season to taste with salt and pepper.

Spoon into a casserole dish and top with cottage cheese. Combine the breadcrumbs, parsley and Parmesan cheese and sprinkle over cottage cheese. Bake for 25 minutes. Serve with jacket potatoes and peas.
Serves 2

Per serve: 1308kJ/311Cals/6.9g fat

# Grilled tuna with potato and celery mash

250g potatoes, peeled and chopped
4 stalks celery, stringed and chopped
1 clove garlic, mashed
1/4 cup skim milk
2 tablespoons non-fat skim milk yoghurt
salt and pepper to taste
2 tuna steaks (about 150g each)
1 carrot, sliced
4 small yellow squash
celery leaves for garnish

Boil or microwave the potato and celery until tender. Drain and place into a bowl with the garlic and mash well. Blend in the milk and yoghurt. Season to taste with salt and pepper. Keep warm.

Grill or sear tuna on a non-stick ridged frypan until cooked to taste. Steam, boil or microwave the carrot and squash until tender. Serve tuna on a bed of potato and celery mash accompanied by the carrots and squash, garnished with celery leaves.
Serves 2

Per serve: 1150kJ/273Cals/7g fat

---

**A simple but delicious marinade for oily fish** (such as mackerel, tuna, swordfish and shark): 1/3 cup light soy sauce, juice of 1/2 a lemon, 1 clove crushed garlic, 1 teaspoon minced ginger, 1 cup pineapple juice.

# Deep sea perch poached in tequila

2 deep sea perch fillets (about 150g each)
1 tablespoon tequila
1/2 teaspoon triple sec liqueur
$1\frac{1}{2}$ tablespoons orange juice
1 teaspoon dill leaf tips
2 teaspoons snipped chives
freshly ground black pepper

Preheat oven to 180°C. Place fish in individual foil parcels. Combine remaining ingredients and spoon over fish. Fold foil up carefully, making sure the tequila mixture can't escape. Bake for 10–15 minutes or until fish is cooked through. Serve with plain boiled potatoes, carrots and peas, with the juices from the parcels spooned over.
Serves 2

Per serve: 562kJ/133Cals/2g fat

---

### Cardinal rule—don't overcook fish

Fish is ready as soon as it loses its translucent appearance and turns opaque all the way through. Overcooking spoils the flavour and texture. To test if fish is cooked, insert a fork into the thickest part of the flesh and gently divide it. It's cooked if it flakes easily. With a whole fish or cutlet, the flesh should come cleanly away from the backbone.

---

# Chilli coriander snapper

Jars of quality chopped fresh ginger, chilli and coriander are handy for those occasions when you're pushed for time, although nothing beats the freshly prepared product.

1/2 teaspoon chopped fresh chilli
1/2 teaspoon chopped fresh coriander
1/4 teaspoon minced ginger
1/2 tablespoon honey
1 tablespoon soy sauce
1/4 cup white wine
2 snapper cutlets (about 150g each)

Combine the chilli, coriander, ginger, honey, soy sauce and white wine in a bowl and mix to combine well. Place the snapper cutlets in a microwave-safe flat dish and pour chilli marinade over. Cover and refrigerate for at least 30 minutes.

Cover the dish with plastic wrap and pierce once to allow steam to escape. Microwave on High (100% power) for $1\frac{1}{2}$–2 minutes. Turn fish over and continue cooking for a further $1\frac{1}{2}$–2 minutes or until the flesh just turns opaque. Serve fish with juices from the dish spooned over, with chat potatoes, yellow zucchini and broccoli. Serves 2

Per serve: 570kJ/135Cals/2g fat

# Swordfish kebabs

300g swordfish fillets, cut into bite-size pieces
4 button mushrooms, halved lengthwise
2 yellow zucchinis, cut into 3cm (1$\frac{1}{4}$") logs
2 green zucchinis, cut into 3cm (1$\frac{1}{4}$") logs
1 small red capsicum, cut into squares
1/4 cup Thai sweet chilli sauce
1/2 tablespoon lemon juice (or to taste)
1/2 tablespoon soy sauce
1/4 teaspoon minced ginger

Thread fish and vegetables alternately onto wooden skewers and place in a flat microwave-safe dish. Combine remaining ingredients and pour over kebabs, brushing or turning to make sure they are well coated. Cover with plastic wrap and marinate for at least 30 minutes.

Pierce plastic wrap once and place dish in the microwave. Cook on High (100% power) for 45 seconds. Turn kebabs over and continue cooking for a further 45 seconds or until fish is just opaque. Serve with steamed rice with dish juices spooned over.
Serves 2

Per serve: 862kJ/205Cals/7g fat

# Piquant prawns

This is another recipe where you can have fun and let your taste buds dictate the flavour. Use your imagination to create your own piquant mixture. However, this one is truly delicious.

500g green prawns, peeled, deveined, tails intact
2 tablespoons lime juice
1 tablespoon Thai sweet chilli sauce
1 clove garlic, crushed
1 tablespoon chopped fresh mint
1/2 tablespoon chopped fresh parsley
salt and pepper to taste

Place the prawns in a microwave-safe dish. Combine remaining ingredients and pour over prawns, stirring to coat well. Cover and cook on High (100% power) for 5 minutes, stirring halfway through cooking. Allow to stand for 3 minutes before serving with steamed rice and a salad.
Serves 2

Per serve: 495kJ/117Cals/1.5g fat

---

### Hints for cooking

*Microwaving:*
- Always cover delicate parts of a whole fish such as the tail with a small strip of foil.
- When microwaving whole fish, thick fillets, cutlets or lobster tail, split the cooking time up and rotate the fish to prevent heat building up in any one part during the cooking time.
- Cook prawns with their tails towards the centre of the dish. Cook for half the required time, turn over and finish cooking.

# Mussels with tomato and garlic

If you don't have a microwave you can still make this recipe by placing all ingredients in a stainless steel saucepan, covering tightly with a lid and cooking over medium heat, shaking pan occasionally, until mussels are all open, about 7 minutes.

1kg mussels in shell
2 spring onions, finely chopped
2 cloves garlic, crushed
2 ripe tomatoes, peeled, seeded and chopped
1/2 cup dry white wine
1 teaspoon chopped fresh basil
cracked black pepper to taste

Scrub and debeard the mussels thoroughly and discard any that stay open when handled. Rinse well. Place in a microwave-safe casserole dish. Combine the remaining ingredients and spoon over the top. Cover tightly with plastic wrap and cook on High (100% power) for 6 minutes, or until mussels just open. If some mussels open before others, remove open ones and keep warm, then continue cooking until all are open. Discard any that don't open.

Spoon mussels into warmed, deep soup bowls and spoon juices from casserole over the top. Serve with crusty bread and a salad.
Serves 2

Per serve: 865kJ/205Cals/2.5g fat

---

- When cooking fillets or cutlets in a sauce or liquid, cook for half the required time, turn over and complete the cooking.
- When microwaving kebabs use bamboo, wooden or microwave skewers (never metal ones). When threading the food onto the skewers, leave a small space between each piece so that they will cook evenly.

# Salmon steaks with cucumber dill sauce

1/4 cup non-fat plain yoghurt
2 tablespoons grated cucumber
2 teaspoons chopped fresh dill (or 1/2 teaspoon dried dill leaf tips)
2 Atlantic salmon cutlets
1 tablespoon lemon juice
freshly grated black pepper

Combine the yoghurt, cucumber and half the dill in a bowl. Cover and set aside. Place the salmon in a microwave-safe dish and sprinkle over the lemon juice, remaining dill and pepper. Cover with plastic wrap and cook on High (100% power) for 2 minutes. Turn cutlets over and continue cooking for a further 2 minutes or until flesh just turns opaque. Serve the salmon with cucumber sauce, boiled potatoes and fresh asparagus.
Serves 2

Per serve: 1195kJ/284Cals/10g fat

# Pearl perch with honey mustard glaze

1 tablespoon dry white wine
1 clove garlic, mashed
1/2 tablespoon Dijon mustard
1 teaspoon honey
1 teaspoon finely chopped fresh parsley
2 pearl perch fillets (about 150g each)

Combine the wine, garlic, mustard, honey and parsley in a small pan and heat gently until combined. Remove from heat. Line a grill pan with foil and place perch on it. Brush the perch with the glaze and cook under a medium heat for 2–3 minutes each side or until just cooked through, brushing with glaze 2–3 times during cooking. Serve with any remaining glaze brushed over, with steamed vegetables and new potatoes.
Serves 2

Per serve: 782kJ/186Cals/2.7g fat

---

*A **simple sauce to go with barbecued fish:*** Combine 1 chopped spring onion, 1 crushed clove garlic, 1 teaspoon chopped fresh tarragon, 1 teaspoon chopped fresh basil, 1 teaspoon snipped chives, and 1 teaspoon chopped fresh parsley. Pour over 2 tablespoons boiling water and allow to stand for 15 minutes before adding 1 tablespoon balsamic vinegar and 1 teaspoon lemon juice. Season to taste with salt and pepper.

# Mediterranean fish casserole

Cut the fish into large pieces because it will shrink during cooking.

2 large ripe tomatoes, peeled, seeded and chopped
1 stalk celery, chopped
1/2 small red capsicum, chopped
4 spring onions, chopped
1 clove garlic, crushed
1 tablespoon red wine
1 tablespoon tomato paste
6 pitted black olives, chopped
1 bay leaf
salt and freshly ground black pepper to taste
300g white fish fillets, cut into pieces
1 teaspoon chopped fresh basil, or 1/4 teaspoon dried (optional)

Place all ingredients, except the fish and basil, in a saucepan and simmer gently for 4–5 minutes. Cool sauce slightly.

Preheat oven to 180°C. Place fish in a casserole dish, sprinkle with basil and pour sauce over. Cover and bake for 15–20 minutes or until fish is cooked through. Serve with spiral pasta and a salad.
Serves 2

Per serve: 1007kJ/239Cals/5.9g fat

# Grilled octopus

300g baby octopus
2 spring onions, finely chopped
1 clove garlic, crushed
1 tablespoon lemon juice
1 teaspoon chopped fresh chilli
1/2 tablespoon soy sauce
1/2 tablespoon fish sauce
1 teaspoon brown sugar
1 teaspoon chopped lemon grass

Wash octopus and pat dry. Place in a bowl with combined remaining ingredients. Cover and marinate for 1 hour. Drain octopus and cook under a very hot grill for 2–3 minutes, turning and basting with marinade as it cooks. Serve with a salad.
Serves 2

Per serve: 542kJ/129Cals/1.85g fat

# Whiting with lemon and dill baste

This is a very simple dish but it's truly delicious as the lemon and dill bring out the delicate flavour of the whiting.

2 whiting fillets (about 150g each)
1 teaspoon chopped fresh dill (or 1/4 teaspoon dried dill leaf tips)
juice of 1/2 lemon
salt and freshly ground black pepper to taste

Preheat oven to 180°C. Place each whiting fillet on a square of foil large enough to form into a parcel. Brush with lemon juice and sprinkle with dill, salt and pepper. Fold foil up into a secure parcel and bake for 20 minutes or until fish is just cooked. Serve with minted new potatoes, peas and carrots.
Serves 2

Per serve: 695kJ/165Cals/2.7g fat

---

*A delightful baste for baked, barbecued or grilled fish:* In a small saucepan combine: 1/4 cup soy sauce, $1\frac{1}{2}$ tablespoons dry sherry, $1\frac{1}{2}$ tablespoons liquid honey, 1 teaspoon grated fresh ginger, 1 crushed clove garlic and pinch dry mustard powder. Heat, stirring until well combined. Use to baste fish before, during and after cooking.

---

## Snapper and vegetable casserole

60g mushrooms, sliced
2 yellow button squash, sliced
1 ripe tomato, peeled, seeded and chopped
2 spring onions, finely chopped
300g snapper fillets, cut into bite-size pieces
salt and ground black pepper to taste
1 cup V8 or tomato juice
1 tablespoon chopped parsley

Preheat oven to 180°C. Layer the vegetables into a casserole dish. Place snapper pieces on top and season with salt and pepper. Pour over V8 or tomato juice and sprinkle with parsley. Bake, uncovered, for about 20 minutes or until fish flakes easily.
Serves 2

Per serve: 908kJ/216Cals/2.7g fat

## Fish with mango and mint

2 white fish fillets (about 150g each)
2 tablespoons dry white wine
1 small mango, peeled and chopped
1 teaspoon chopped fresh mint

Preheat oven to 180°C. Place the fish on a square of foil large enough to fold up into a parcel. Sprinkle over the wine, mango pieces and mint. Fold foil into a parcel and bake for 20 minutes or until fish flakes easily. Serve with steamed vegetables and baby potatoes.
Serves 2

Per serve: 870kJ/207Cals/2.7g fat

# Seafood stir-fry

This is one of my daughter Lisby's recipes. It is very quick and easy to prepare and its flavour belies its low-fat content.

1 calamari hood
6 scallops
6 green prawns, peeled and deveined
2 tablespoons soy sauce (salt-reduced)
2 tablespoons Thai sweet chilli sauce
1–2 bok choy (depending on size)
1 small red capsicum, cut into long strips
2 cups hot cooked long grain rice

Cut calamari hood into rectangles about 3cm x 5cm, then score one side in a diamond pattern. Place all seafood in a bowl. Add soy sauce and sweet chilli sauce and mix well. Cover and marinade for 30 minutes. Heat non-stick wok. (If not non-stick add a teaspoon of olive oil.) Stir-fry seafood and marinade in wok for 2–3 minutes. Add bok choy and capsicum and stir-fry for a further minute or so, until bok choy begins to wilt. Serve hot over boiled rice.
Serves 2

Per serve: 1400kJ/333Cals/2.6g fat

# 14  Pasta and rice

## Quick tuna and tomato pasta

This is ideal for those days when you get home from work and can hardly bear the idea of cooking—but still want something satisfying to eat.

425g peeled Italian tomatoes
1 clove garlic, crushed
2 anchovy fillets, drained on paper towel
1/2 tablespoon capers
3 stuffed olives, sliced
210g can tuna, packed in brine
1/2 teaspoon dried mixed herbs
freshly ground pepper to taste
2 cups hot cooked pasta
2 tablespoons finely chopped fresh parsley

Puree the tomatoes in a processor, or place in a saucepan and mash with a wooden spoon. Add the garlic, anchovies, capers, olives, tuna and mixed herbs. Season to taste with pepper. Simmer gently for 10–15 minutes until the sauce reduces and thickens. The time will depend on the juiciness of the tomatoes. Serve sauce spooned over hot, cooked pasta, sprinkled with parsley.
Serves 2

Per serve: 1429kJ/340Cals/6.35g fat

# Beans with rice and vegetables

1/2 cup brown rice
1 carrot, chopped
1 onion, peeled and chopped
1 clove garlic, crushed
1 teaspoon ground cumin
1/2 teaspoon turmeric
1/2 teaspoon ground ginger
1/4 teaspoon chilli powder
1 cup chicken stock
1 tablespoon lemon juice
210g can red kidney beans, drained
salt and pepper to taste

Place the rice, carrot, onion, garlic, spices and stock in a saucepan. Bring to the boil, stirring constantly. Cover and simmer for about 40 minutes or until rice is cooked. Stir in the lemon juice and beans and season to taste with salt and pepper. Continue cooking, uncovered, until beans are heated through and all liquid has been absorbed. Serve with crusty bread and a green salad.
Serves 2

Per serve: 1312kJ/312Cals/1.75g fat

# Savoury rice with vegetables

1 medium onion, chopped
1 clove garlic, crushed
1/4 cup dry white wine
1/2 cup Calrose rice
1 carrot, peeled and diced
1 stalk celery, chopped
1 cup chicken stock
1/2 teaspoon Italian mixed herbs
salt and pepper to taste
1/4 cup corn kernels
1/4 cup peas
2 tablespoons grated Parmesan cheese
2 tablespoons chopped parsley

In a medium saucepan, simmer the onion and garlic in wine until softened. Stir in rice, carrot, celery, stock and mixed herbs. Season to taste with salt and pepper. Cover and simmer, stirring occasionally, for 10 minutes.

Add corn and peas. Continue cooking for a further 10 minutes or until rice and vegetables are tender. Serve with Parmesan and parsley.

*Note:* Check the amount of liquid in the pan—by the end of cooking all the liquid should have been absorbed by the rice; if you think that it is drying out too quickly add a little more stock; if you think it will be runny, then remove lid and stir with a chopstick to evaporate excess liquid.
Serves 2

Per serve: 1310kJ/312Cals/2.62g fat

# Rice with crab and corn

1 small leek, washed and chopped
1 clove garlic, crushed
1/3 cup dry white wine
1/2 cup Calrose rice
1 stalk celery, chopped
1/2 small red capsicum, diced
1 teaspoon dried dill leaf tips
210g can crab meat, drained, liquid reserved
chicken stock
1/2 cup corn kernels
salt and pepper to taste
2 tablespoons Parmesan cheese
2 tablespoons chopped parsley

In a medium sized saucepan, simmer the leek and garlic in the wine until the leek has softened. Stir in the rice, celery, capsicum and dill. Make up the drained crab juices to 1 cup with chicken stock. Add to pan, stirring well. Cover and simmer for 10 minutes.

Add the crab meat and corn and season to taste with salt and pepper. Cover and continue cooking for a further 10 minutes or until rice is plump and tender. Serve with Parmesan and parsley sprinkled over.

*Note:* Check the amount of liquid in the pan—by the end of cooking all the liquid should have been absorbed by the rice; if you think that it is drying out too quickly add a little more stock; if you think it will be runny, then remove lid and stir with a chopstick to evaporate excess liquid.
Serves 2

Per serve: 1659kJ/395Cals/3.5g fat

# Seafood rice salad

1 cup cold cooked long grain rice
1/4 cup extra light sour cream
1/4 cup non-fat yoghurt
1/2 tablespoon lemon juice
pinch chilli powder
salt and pepper to taste
6 cooked king prawns, peeled, deveined, cut into bite-size pieces
6 marinated scallops, drained
6 marinated mussels, drained
1 stalk celery, chopped
1/2 small red capsicum, chopped
1/4 cup corn kernels

Place the rice in a large bowl. Combine the sour cream, yoghurt, lemon juice and chilli powder and season to taste with salt and pepper. Pour over rice and carefully blend through using a fork or two chopsticks so you don't mash the rice. Add all remaining ingredients and mix through. Serve with cherry tomatoes and a green salad.
Serves 2

Per serve: 1659kJ/395Cals/8.9g fat

# Beef with snow peas and rice

250g rump steak, trimmed of all fat, cut into thin strips
1 small onion, cut into petals
1 clove garlic, crushed
1/4 teaspoon chopped fresh chilli
1/4 cup beef stock
30g snow peas, topped and tailed
1 1/2 cups cooked long grain rice
1/2 tablespoon hoi sin sauce
1/2 tablespoon Thai sweet chilli sauce

Heat a non-stick wok or frypan over medium high heat and quickly stir-fry the steak until it changes colour—this will only take a minute or so. Remove from the pan with a slotted spoon. Add the onion, garlic, chilli and stock to the pan and simmer, stirring, until the onion is tender.

Add the snow peas and continue cooking for a further 2–3 minutes or until snow peas turn bright green. Return meat to the pan with the rice and sauces and toss for 3–4 minutes or until rice is heated through. Serve with soy sauce, if liked.
Serves 2

Per serve: 1311kJ/312Cals/4.5g fat

# Capsicum stuffed with beef and mushrooms

Choose squarish capsicums that will sit well on their bottoms.

2 red capsicums
2 spring onions, chopped
1 clove garlic, crushed
1/4 cup beef stock
250g rump steak, minced
60g mushrooms, chopped
2 ripe tomatoes, peeled, seeded and chopped
salt and pepper to taste
1/2 cup cooked long grain rice

Preheat oven to 180°C. Slice the tops from the capsicums and retain. Remove seeds and veins from inside the capsicums and wash and pat dry with paper towel.

Simmer the spring onions and garlic in the beef stock until softened. Add the mince, mushrooms and tomatoes and season to taste with salt and pepper. Cook, stirring, until mince changes colour. Remove from the heat and stir through the rice. Stuff the capsicums with this mixture, replace tops and place in a baking dish. Bake for 20–30 minutes or until capsicums are tender. Serve with a salad and crusty bread.
Serves 2

Per serve: 1111kJ/264Cals/4g fat

# Rice with chickpeas and corn

This is good as a no-meat dish on its own, or as an accompaniment to lamb or pork.

2 spring onions, chopped
1 small clove garlic (optional), crushed
1/4 cup white wine
1/2 cup long grain rice
1 cup chicken stock
salt and pepper to taste
1/2 cup cooked chickpeas
1/4 cup corn kernels
1/4 cup frozen green peas
2 tablespoons chopped fresh parsley

Simmer the spring onions and garlic in the wine, in a medium saucepan, until softened. Stir in the rice and chicken stock. Season to taste with salt and pepper. Cover and simmer for 10 minutes. Add the chickpeas, corn and peas and stir through rice. Cover and continue to cook for a further 5 minutes or until rice is tender. Serve sprinkle with chopped fresh parsley and crusty wholemeal bread, or spoon into pita pockets.
Serves 2

Per serve: 1994kJ/296.5Cals/1.18g fat

# Chicken and mushroom risotto

1 onion, chopped
1 clove garlic, crushed
1/4 cup white wine
1½ cups chicken stock (approx.)
1/3 cup arborio rice
250g chicken breast fillets, trimmed of all fat, sliced
1/2 teaspoon Italian mixed herbs
salt and pepper to taste
60g mushrooms, sliced
1/4 cup corn kernels
2 tablespoons Parmesan cheese
2 tablespoons chopped fresh parsley

Simmer the onion and garlic in a saucepan with the white wine until onion has softened. Have the stock just at simmer point in another pan. Add rice to onions and stir well. Add 1/4 cup of stock and cook, stirring, until rice absorbs the stock. Stir in the chicken and mixed herbs, salt, pepper and another 1/4 cup of stock and continue to stir until chicken changes colour and the stock is absorbed. Add the mushrooms and corn and more stock. Continue in this way until the rice is plump and tender but still with a bite to it. You may or may not need all the stock. Serve sprinkled with Parmesan cheese and parsley.
Serves 2

Per serve: 1508kJ/338Cals/5.5g fat

# Ham, mushroom and zucchini pasta

1 onion, chopped
1 clove garlic, crushed
1/4 cup white wine
50g lean ham, cut into strips
60g mushrooms, sliced
1 large zucchini, sliced
1 large ripe tomato, peeled, seeded and chopped
1/8 teaspoon oregano
salt and pepper to taste
2 cups hot cooked pasta
2 tablespoons chopped parsley

Simmer the onion and garlic in a saucepan with the wine until onion has softened. Add the ham, mushrooms, zucchini, tomato, oregano and salt and pepper to taste. Cover and simmer gently for 4–5 minutes or until mushrooms are soft.

Toss sauce through hot pasta. Serve immediately, sprinkled with parsley.
Serves 2

Per serve: 1237kJ/294Cals/3.5g fat

# Pasta with chicken livers

Chicken livers are full of iron and 100g contains only 6g fat, so I think they are well worth including occasionally in the diet, especially when other red meats are being reduced.

1 onion, finely chopped
1 clove garlic, crushed
1/4 cup white wine
100g chicken livers, washed, trimmed and cut into bite-size pieces
1 tablespoon brandy
2 ripe tomatoes, peeled, seeded and chopped
60g mushrooms, chopped
1/2 teaspoon Italian mixed herbs
2 cups hot cooked pasta
2 tablespoons chopped parsley

Simmer the onion and garlic in a saucepan with the wine until the onion has softened. Stir in the livers and brandy and cook, stirring, until the livers change colour. Add the tomatoes, mushrooms and herbs, stir well, then cover and simmer for 5 minutes. Toss sauce through hot cooked pasta and serve sprinkled with chopped parsley.
Serves 2

Per serve: 1499kJ/356Cals/4g fat

# Guilt-free spaghetti bolognese

1 onion, chopped
1 clove garlic, crushed
3/4 cup beef stock
250g rump steak, trimmed of all fat, minced
2 ripe tomatoes, peeled, seeded and chopped
1 tablespoon tomato paste
1/4 teaspoon dried Italian mixed herbs
salt and pepper to taste
60g mushrooms, sliced
2 cups hot cooked spaghetti
1 tablespoon Parmesan cheese
2 tablespoons chopped fresh parsley

Simmer the onion and garlic in a saucepan with 1/4 cup beef stock until onion has softened. Add the mince and cook, stirring, until it changes colour, breaking any lumps up with a wooden spoon. Add the tomatoes, tomato paste, herbs and salt and pepper to taste. Cover and simmer gently for 20–30 minutes or until meat is tender. Five minutes before the end of cooking add the mushrooms.

Place hot spaghetti into warm serving bowls, spoon sauce over and serve sprinkled with Parmesan cheese and parsley.
Serves 2

Per serve: 1736kJ/429Cals/4.8g fat

# Zucchini, capsicum and sour cream pasta

1 onion, chopped
1 clove garlic, crushed
1/2 cup white wine
1 ripe tomato, peeled, seeded and chopped
1/2 cup small broccoli florets
1 stalk celery, chopped
1 zucchini, sliced
1/2 small red capsicum, diced
1/2 teaspoon Italian mixed herbs
salt and pepper to taste
100g extra light sour cream
2 cups hot cooked pasta
2 tablespoons chopped fresh parsley

Simmer the onion and garlic in a saucepan with 1/4 cup wine until onion has softened. Add vegetables, herbs and remaining wine, and season to taste with salt and pepper. Cover and simmer for 5 minutes or until vegetables are tender crisp. Lower heat to minimum and stir in sour cream to just heat through—too high a heat will make the sour cream separate. Toss sauce through hot pasta. Serve sprinkled with parsley.
Serves 2

Per serve: 1550kJ/369Cals/3.5g fat

# Tuna, mushroom and artichoke pasta

1 onion, chopped
1 clove garlic, crushed
1/2 cup chicken stock
60g mushrooms, sliced
1/2 tablespoon lemon juice
185g can tuna in spring water or brine, drained and flaked
2 large canned artichokes, drained and quartered
salt and pepper to taste
100g extra light sour cream
2 cups hot cooked pasta
1 teaspoon grated lemon zest

Simmer the onion and garlic in a saucepan with 1/4 cup stock until onion has softened. Add the mushrooms, lemon juice and remaining stock and continue cooking until mushrooms soften. Stir in the tuna, artichokes and season to taste with salt and pepper. Cover and cook for 3–4 minutes or until heated through. Turn heat to low and stir through the sour cream so that it just warms through. Place hot pasta into warmed serving bowls. Top with tuna sauce and sprinkle with lemon zest.
Serves 2

Per serve: 1834kJ/436Cals/4.1g fat

# Chicken meatballs with pasta

250g chicken breast fillet, minced
2 spring onions, very finely chopped
2 tablespoons dry breadcrumbs
1 teaspoon dried coriander leaves
salt and freshly ground pepper to taste
1 egg white
1 onion, chopped
1 clove garlic, crushed
1/4 cup white wine
1/4 cup tomato puree
1 cup chicken stock
1 teaspoon Worcestershire sauce
1 teaspoon Italian mixed herbs
2 cups hot cooked pasta

Combine the mince, spring onions, breadcrumbs, coriander, salt, pepper and egg white and mix well. With wet hands, form mince into small balls the size of a walnut. Place on a plate, cover and refrigerate while you make the sauce.

Simmer the onion and garlic in a saucepan with the wine until onion has softened. Add the tomato puree, stock, Worcestershire sauce and herbs. Stir well. Cover and simmer for 10–15 minutes.

Drop meatballs into simmering sauce and cook, stirring occasionally, for 10–15 minutes or until meatballs are cooked through.

Place hot cooked pasta into warmed serving bowls. Spoon sauce and meatballs over and serve.
Serves 2

Per serve: 1840kJ/438Cals/4.5g fat

# Tomato, anchovy and olive pasta

The brine-packed olives in this dish give you the flavour without excess fat kilojoules.

1 onion, finely chopped
1 clove garlic, crushed
1/4 cup chicken stock
1 large ripe tomato, peeled, seeded and chopped
6 anchovy fillets, drained on paper towel, chopped
1/4 cup red wine
6 pitted black olives (packed in brine), chopped
freshly ground pepper to taste
2 cups hot cooked pasta
2 tablespoons chopped fresh parsley

Simmer the onion and garlic in a saucepan with the stock until onion has softened. Stir in the tomato, anchovies, wine and olives, and season to taste with pepper—with the anchovies and olives you probably won't need salt. Cover and simmer gently for 10–15 minutes.

Place hot cooked pasta into warm serving bowls. Spoon sauce over and serve sprinkled with parsley.
Serves 2

Per serve: 1325kJ/315Cals/5.5g fat

# Pasta with ham and avocado

1/2 small avocado, mashed
1 clove garlic, crushed
1/2 tablespoon chilli sauce
1 teaspoon lemon juice
pinch chilli powder
2 slices lean leg ham, cut into strips
4 cherry tomatoes, halved
1/2 tablespoon snipped chives
freshly ground pepper to taste
2 cups hot cooked pasta
2 tablespoons chopped fresh parsley

Combine all ingredients except pasta and parsley. Toss avocado sauce and pasta together. Serve in warm pasta bowls sprinkled with parsley.
Serves 2

Per serve: 1207kJ/287Cals/7.5g fat

# Pasta with spinach and pine nut sauce

250g block frozen chopped spinach, thawed
60g mushrooms, sliced
1/2 tablespoon lemon juice
freshly ground black pepper to taste
100g extra light sour cream
2 cups hot cooked pasta
1/2 tablespoon pine nuts

Place the spinach, mushrooms, lemon juice and pepper in a small saucepan, cover and simmer until mushrooms are soft and moisture has mostly evaporated from the spinach. Reduce heat to low and stir through sour cream to just warm through.

Place hot cooked pasta into warm bowls and top with spinach and mushroom sauce sprinkled with pine nuts.
Serves 2

Per serve: 1400kJ/333Cals/5.75g fat

# Pasta with artichokes, sun-dried tomatoes and chilli

This is another of my daughter Lisby's recipes. It is extremely easy to prepare but truly delicious.

6 sun-dried tomatoes (dry-packed), chopped
6 canned artichoke hearts, drained, roughly chopped
1 teaspoon olive oil
1 fresh chilli, seeded and roughly chopped
ground dried chilli flakes to taste
salt and pepper to taste
2 cups hot cooked spiral pasta
1 tablespoon grated Parmesan cheese
2 tablespoons chopped parsley

Place the sun-dried tomatoes in a small bowl and pour boiling water over to just cover. Stand 10 minutes. Drain, reserving soaking liquid.

Slowly heat a non-stick saucepan. Add artichokes and oil, stir for 1 minute. Add sun-dried tomatoes, chilli and chilli flakes, and season to taste with salt and pepper. Stir until heated through. If mixture seems a little dry add a little of the tomato-soaking liquid. Toss hot cooked pasta through artichoke mixture. Sprinkle with grated cheese and parsley and serve with crusty bread and a mixed green salad.
Serves 2

Per serve:1187kJ/282Cals/4.5g fat

# 15 Vegetable dishes

## Artichokes with spicy yoghurt dip

2 globe artichokes
lemon juice
200g non-fat skim milk yoghurt
1 clove garlic
2 tablespoons honey
2 teaspoons minced chilli
1 teaspoon minced ginger
ground black pepper to taste
2 tablespoons chopped fresh parsley

Slice stems from artichokes. Remove and discard coarse outer leaves and slice off the top third of the globe. Snip away any remaining thorny leaf tips. Place end up in 3cm boiling water to which a little lemon juice has been added. Cover with a lid and simmer for 20–25 minutes or until stem end is tender. Drain.

Combine remaining ingredients and chill until ready to serve. Serve yoghurt dip with hot artichokes.
Serves 2

Per serve: 685kJ/163Cals/0.25g fat

# Tomato, bean and mushroom casserole

This makes a very generous serving for two people, but as it freezes well you can store any leftovers for another occasion.

1 small onion, sliced
1 small clove garlic, crushed
1 small tomato, peeled and chopped
60g green beans, sliced
60g mushrooms, sliced
60g corn kernels
1 small carrot, sliced
1 small zucchini, sliced
1 cup water
2 tablespoons tomato paste
1 teaspoon ground cumin
1/2 teaspoon dried basil
dash Worcestershire sauce
salt and pepper to taste

Place all ingredients in a heavy-based saucepan and simmer gently until vegetables are cooked, about 20 minutes. Serve with couscous and a green salad.
Serves 2

Per serve: 360kJ/85Cals/0.45g fat

# Mixed vegetable pasta bake

1 clove garlic, crushed
2 spring onions, chopped
1 large carrot, chopped
1/4 cup chicken or vegetable stock
1 cup V8 or tomato juice
1 tablespoon tomato paste
1/2 teaspoon chopped fresh tarragon
1 zucchini, cut into 3cm slices
1 large potato, cooked and diced
1 cup cooked spiral or elbow pasta
nutmeg to taste
60g grated reduced-fat tasty cheese
1 tablespoon chopped fresh parsley

Place the garlic, onions and carrots in a heatproof casserole dish with the stock. Simmer over gentle heat for 5–6 minutes. Add the V8 or tomato juice, tomato paste, tarragon and zucchini. Simmer 4–5 minutes. Stir in the potato, pasta and nutmeg. Sprinkle over combined cheese and parsley. Bake at 180°C for 10 to 15 minutes or until golden brown and heated through. Serve with crusty multigrain bread and a green salad.
Serves 2 (with hearty appetites)

Per serve: 1365kJ/325Cals/5.75g fat

# Pasta with mushrooms and beans

1/2 cup chicken or vegetable stock
2 spring onions, chopped
1/2 small red capsicum, seeded and chopped
1 stalk celery, chopped
1 clove garlic, crushed
1/4 teaspoon dried oregano
1/4 teaspoon dried basil
black pepper to taste
100g mushrooms, sliced
210g can red kidney beans, rinsed and drained
2 tablespoons tomato paste
1 cup water
2 cups hot cooked pasta
2 tablespoons grated Parmesan cheese
finely chopped parsley for garnish

Place the stock in a saucepan with the onions, capsicum, celery, garlic, oregano and basil. Season to taste with pepper. Simmer gently, stirring occasionally, for 4–5 minutes. Add the mushrooms, beans, tomato paste and water. Stir well. Simmer for a further 10 minutes until sauce thickens slightly. If sauce seems a little thin, you can thicken it with some cornflour mixed to a paste with a little water. Stir until mixture boils and thickens. Serve over cooked pasta sprinkled with Parmesan cheese and parsley.
Serves 2

Per serve: 1345kJ/320Cals/3.7g fat

# Tomato and artichoke pasta sauce

1/4 cup chicken or vegetable stock or white wine
2 spring onions, chopped
1 clove garlic, crushed
425g can peeled tomatoes, chopped
1 tablespoon chopped fresh basil
1 tablespoon chopped fresh parsley
200g marinated artichoke hearts, drained and quartered
2 cups hot cooked pasta
2 tablespoons grated Parmesan cheese

Place the stock or wine in a saucepan with the onions and garlic and simmer for 3–4 minutes. Stir in the tomatoes, basil and parsley. Bring to the boil, reduce heat and simmer, uncovered, for about 20 minutes until sauce reduces and thickens. Add the artichoke hearts and simmer until heated through. Serve over cooked pasta, sprinkled with Parmesan cheese.
Serves 2

Per serve: 1336kJ/318Cals/3.1g fat

# Hearty vegetable soup

This is a wonderfully satisfying soup which is quick to make. Eat it for your evening meal with some lovely crusty bread and you'll feel content and satisfied afterwards. The carbohydrate is very calming and it contains no fat. This soup also freezes well, so it's well worth making a large batch so you can have some on standby in the freezer.

1.5 litres chicken or vegetable stock
1 large potato, peeled and chopped
3 carrots, peeled and chopped
1 small turnip, peeled and chopped
2 stalks celery, chopped
1 large onion, peeled and chopped
1 clove garlic, crushed
2 tomatoes, peeled, seeded and chopped
4 spinach leaves, washed and shredded
10 green beans, topped, tailed and sliced
1/2 teaspoon dried mixed herbs
salt and pepper to taste

Place all ingredients in a large saucepan. Bring to the boil, skim off any scum that rises to the surface, reduce heat and simmer until all the vegetables are tender—about 20–25 minutes. You can serve the soup as it is or blended until smooth. Serve with a dollop of non-fat yoghurt if liked, sprinkled with chopped fresh parsley.
Serves 8

Per serve: 283kJ/67Cals/0g fat

# Iced lettuce and cucumber soup

1 litre chicken or vegetable stock
1 iceberg lettuce, washed
1 cucumber, sliced
1 tablespoon lemon juice
pinch grated nutmeg
1 teaspoon chopped fresh tarragon
salt and pepper to taste

Place the stock, lettuce, cucumber, lemon juice and nutmeg in a large pan. Bring to the boil, skim off any scum that rises to the surface. Reduce heat and simmer for 10–15 minutes. Puree soup until smooth. Stir through the tarragon and season to taste with salt and pepper. Chill well. Serve soup with a dollop of non-fat yoghurt and chopped parsley, if liked.
Serves 4

Per serve: 128kJ/30Cals/0g fat

# Microwave jacket potatoes

2 large potatoes, about 250g each

Scrub potatoes well, rinse and pierce in several places with a skewer. Place on paper towel on the turntable. Microwave on High (100% power) for 4 minutes. Turn potatoes over and continue cooking for a further 3–4 minutes. Wrap in foil (or a clean tea-towel if you have no foil) and allow to stand for 5 minutes.
Serves 2

Per serve: 730kJ/175Cals/0g fat

# Hearty pumpkin soup

This soup is very quick to prepare, and makes a satisfying lunch or supper dish accompanied by crusty multigrain bread. It freezes well, so make a batch and freeze in individual serving sizes to have on hand when hunger strikes and you're looking for something tasty and filling.

750g pumpkin, peeled, seeded and chopped
1 large potato, peeled and chopped
1 large onion, chopped
1 clove garlic, crushed
2 stalks celery, chopped
1 litre chicken or vegetable stock
salt and pepper to taste
freshly grated nutmeg

Place prepared vegetables in a large saucepan and cover with stock. Season to taste with salt and pepper. Bring to the boil, skim off any scum which rises to the top. Reduce heat and simmer for 20–25 minutes or until vegetables are tender. Puree by processing in a blender or pushing through a sieve. Season with freshly grated nutmeg. Serve with a dollop of non-fat yoghurt and snipped chives or chopped parsley, if liked.
Serves 4

Per serve: 675kJ/160Cals/0g fat

# Black beans, capsicum and coriander

1 small onion, chopped
1 clove garlic, crushed
1/4 cup white wine
1 small red capsicum, chopped
1/4 cup orange juice
1 tablespoon lime juice
1/4 teaspoon cayenne pepper (or to taste)
1/4 small, slightly under-ripe pawpaw, peeled, seeded and chopped
1 teaspoon chopped fresh coriander
150g canned black beans, drained and rinsed
1 cup cooked long grain rice

Simmer the onion and garlic in the wine until onion has softened. Add the capsicum, orange and lime juice and cayenne pepper. Simmer for 5 minutes or until capsicum is tender. Add the pawpaw and coriander. Cook for 1 minute, then stir in the beans and continue to simmer for a further 5 minutes or until heated through. Serve with cooked rice.
Serves 2

Per serve: 1744kJ/415cals/1.5g fat

# Marinated tofu and vegetables

125g firm tofu, cubed
1 tablespoon tomato sauce
1 tablespoon fish sauce
1 tablespoon lemon juice
1 tablespoon brown sugar
1 tablespoon snipped chives
1 teaspoon chopped fresh chilli
1 teaspoon chopped fresh coriander
1/4 cup broccoli florets
1/4 cup cauliflower florets
1 small carrot, sliced diagonally
1/2 small red capsicum, chopped
1 cup hot cooked long grain rice
1 tablespoon chopped fresh parsley

Place the tofu in a bowl. Combine the tomato sauce, fish sauce, lemon juice, sugar, chives, chilli and coriander. Cover and marinate for 1 hour. Remove tofu with a slotted spoon and set aside. Pour marinade into a non-stick wok. Bring to a simmer and add vegetables. Cook until vegetables are tender crisp. Add tofu and heat through. Serve with rice, sprinkled with parsley.
Serves 2

Per serve: 976kJ/232Cals/4.5g fat

# Mixed vegetable parcels

1 small onion, finely chopped
1 clove garlic, finely chopped
1/4 cup white wine
1 small carrot, diced finely
1/4 cup chopped red capsicum
1 small bok choy, chopped
1 egg, beaten
1/2 tablespoon Parmesan cheese
salt and pepper to taste
2 sheets filo pastry
skim milk
poppy seeds

Simmer the onion and garlic in the wine in a non-stick frypan until tender. Add the remaining vegetables and stir-fry until tender crisp. Cool. Stir in combined egg, Parmesan cheese and salt and pepper to taste.

Preheat oven to 190°C. Working with one sheet of pastry at a time, brush with milk and fold in half. Place half the vegetable mixture down centre of pastry, brush pastry with milk and fold up into a neat parcel, brushing with milk at each fold. Repeat with remaining pastry and filling. Place on a non-stick baking tray. Brush with milk and sprinkle with poppy seeds. Bake for 25–30 minutes or until pastry is golden brown. Serve with salad.
Serves 2

Per serve: 633kJ/150Cals/3.8g fat

## Spicy chickpeas and potatoes

1 small onion, chopped
1 clove garlic, crushed
1/4 cup white wine
1 tablespoon tomato paste
1 tablespoon water
375g canned chickpeas
1 large potato, peeled and chopped
1/2 cup vegetable stock
1/2 teaspoon ground cumin
1/4 teaspoon chopped fresh chilli
dash Tabasco sauce
1/2 tablespoon lemon juice

Simmer the onion and garlic in the wine in a saucepan until onion is tender. Stir in remaining ingredients, cover and simmer for 20 minutes. Serve with tortillas, if liked.
Serves 2

Per serve: 1187kJ/282Cals/4g fat

## Chickpea and vegetable curry

375g can chickpeas, drained
1 onion, chopped
1 clove garlic, crushed
1/2 small red capsicum, chopped
1/2 small green capsicum, chopped
300g Indian tikka masala cooking sauce

Combine all ingredients in a saucepan and simmer gently for 25–30 minutes. Serve with steamed rice, side dishes of banana and lemon juice, tomato and onion, cucumber and yoghurt, mango chutney and microwaved pappadums (see page 185).
Serves 2

Per serve: 1155kJ/275Cals/5.5g fat

# Potatoes with chilli beans

This is ideal for those occasions when you're starving and want a satisfying meal fast.

2 Desiree or other baking potatoes, about 250g each
1/2 cup three bean mix (or baked beans), drained
1 tablespoon tomato paste
1 tablespoon chilli sauce
1/2 teaspoon chilli powder (or to taste)
1 tablespoon snipped chives
2 tablespoons non-fat yoghurt

Scrub potatoes and pierce two or three times with a skewer. Place on a sheet of paper towel on the turntable of your microwave. Microwave for 7 minutes on High (100% power), turning over halfway through cooking. Remove from microwave and wrap in foil. Allow to stand for 5 minutes.

Meanwhile, heat beans, tomato paste, chilli sauce, chilli powder and chives together in a small saucepan or in the microwave. When potatoes are ready, place onto warmed serving plates and cut in half. Fill with chilli beans and serve with a dollop of yoghurt.
Serves 2

Per serve: 1775kJ/422Cals/0.5g fat

# Vegetable stir-fry with almonds

1 small onion, chopped
1 clove garlic, crushed
1/4 cup white wine
1 bok choy, chopped
1 small carrot, sliced diagonally
1/2 small red capsicum, chopped
1 stalk celery, chopped
1 tablespoon oyster sauce
1 tablespoon soy sauce (salt-reduced)
30g toasted almonds, chopped
2 cups hot cooked rice

Heat a non-stick wok over medium high heat. Stir-fry the onion and garlic in the white wine until tender. Increase heat to high and add the vegetables. Stir-fry vegetables until bright in colour and tender crisp. Add the oyster and soy sauces and almonds, tossing until heated through. Serve with steamed rice.
Serves 2

Per serve: 1069kJ/254Cals/0.5g fat

Nuts and seeds can be the downfall of many low-fat diets, not only nibbled with drinks but also used in recipes. Although nuts and seeds are nutritious food, they are also energy dense—that is, they are high in kilojoules and fat compared to their weight. Where you see nuts used in a recipe either omit them or use half the amount and chop them finely—you will still get the flavour without all the kilojoules.

# Vegetarian bolognese sauce

1 small onion, chopped
1 small clove garlic, crushed
1/4 cup vegetable stock
210g can peeled tomatoes
1 tablespoon tomato paste
1 stalk celery, chopped
1 small carrot, chopped
1/4 cup red wine
1/2 teaspoon dried Italian mixed herbs
salt and freshly ground black pepper to taste
125g mushrooms, chopped
2 cups hot cooked pasta

Simmer the onion and garlic in a saucepan with the vegetable stock until onion has softened. Stir in remaining ingredients except mushrooms and pasta. Simmer for 15 minutes. Add the mushrooms and continue cooking for a further 5 minutes. Serve with pasta of choice, crusty bread and salad.
Serves 2

Per serve: 1180/280Cals/0.25g fat

# Tomato, corn and pea curry

1 teaspoon turmeric
1 teaspoon ground cumin
1 teaspoon ground coriander
1/4 teaspoon chilli powder
1 small onion, chopped
1 clove garlic, crushed
1/4 cup white wine
1 bay leaf
2 tomatoes, peeled, seeded and chopped
1/4 cup corn kernels
1/4 cup frozen peas, thawed
150ml vegetable stock
salt and freshly ground pepper to taste
2 cups hot cooked rice

Dry-fry the spices in a non-stick saucepan over gentle heat, stirring occasionally, until aromatic. Add the onion and garlic with the wine and simmer until onion has softened. Add remaining ingredients, except rice, and simmer for 10–15 minutes. Serve with rice and side dishes of mango chutney, microwaved pappadums, cucumber and yoghurt and tomatoes and chopped onion.
Serves 2

Per serve: 1160kJ/276Cals/0.1g fat

---

### Microwaved pappadums

You can save over 22g fat by microwaving pappadums instead of frying them. Simply place a sheet of paper towel on the turntable, place pappadums in a single layer on top, cover with another sheet of paper towel and microwave for 30 seconds. 100g fried pappadums = 22.7g fat; 100g microwaved pappadums = 0.4g fat!

---

# Cracked wheat and tomato salad

50g cracked wheat
2/3 cup boiling water
1/4 cup chopped red capsicum
1/4 cup chopped cucumber
1 tablespoon lemon juice
2 tablespoons chopped fresh parsley
2 tablespoons chopped fresh mint
1 large tomato, peeled, seeded and chopped
salt and pepper to taste
mixed salad greens

Soak the wheat in the water for 20 minutes or until the grains have swollen and absorbed the water. Stir through remaining ingredients. Cover and refrigerate for 30 minutes for flavours to mingle. Serve with salad greens and crusty bread.
Serves 2

Per serve: 405kJ/96Cals/0.4g fat

# Millet, bean and capsicum pilaf

1 onion, chopped
1 clove garlic, crushed
1/4 cup white wine or vegetable stock
1 carrot, chopped
1 stalk celery, chopped
1/2 small red capsicum, chopped
210g can three bean mix
2 ripe tomatoes, peeled, seeded and chopped
1/4 teaspoon dried mixed herbs
salt and pepper to taste
80g millet
300ml water

Simmer the onion and garlic in a saucepan with the wine until onion has softened. Add the carrot, celery, capsicum, beans, tomatoes, herbs and salt and pepper to taste. Cover and simmer for 15–20 minutes.

Meanwhile, place the millet in a saucepan and dry-fry, stirring constantly, over medium heat for about 5 minutes. Add the water, cover and simmer for 15–20 minutes or until millet is cooked and fluffy. Place millet in a serving bowl and top with vegetables and beans.
Serves 2

Per serve: 1385kJ/329Cals/1.37g fat

# 16 Salad dressings, sauces, salsas and chutneys

## Creamy salad dressing

If this dressing is too thick (yoghurt comes in different densities), thin it with a little skim milk.

200g non-fat skim milk yoghurt
1 Lebanese cucumber, peeled, seeded and chopped
1 clove garlic, crushed
1 tablespoon lemon juice
1 tablespoon chopped parsley
freshly ground black pepper to taste

Combine all ingredients.
Makes about 1½ cups

Per 1/4 cup: 96kJ/23Cals/neg fat

## Curried yoghurt dressing

This gives a rice salad a real lift. Add some chopped tomatoes, cucumber, cooked peas and cashews and you'll have a tasty, nutritious meal.

200g non-fat skim milk yoghurt
1 teaspoon curry powder
1 teaspoon freshly squeezed lemon juice

Combine all ingredients. Refrigerate until ready to serve.
Makes about 3/4 cup

Per 1/4 cup: 180kJ/43Cals/neg. fat

## Creamy horseradish dressing

This adds a lovely 'bite' to salad greens, especially when served with lean steak.

100g non-fat skim milk yoghurt
2 tablespoons grated horseradish
freshly ground black pepper to taste

Combine all ingredients. Toss through mixed salad greens.
Makes about 3/4 cup

Per 1/4 cup: 83kJ/20Cals/neg fat


## Lemon Dijon dressing

This is lovely with a chicken salad.

100g non-fat skim milk yoghurt
2 tablespoons lemon juice
1 tablespoon Dijon mustard
1/2 teaspoon dried tarragon
freshly ground black pepper

Combine all ingredients. Cover and chill for 30 minutes to allow flavours to develop.
Makes about 3/4 cup

Per 1/4 cup: 100kJ/24Cals/neg

# Sesame soy garlic dressing

1/2 cup rice vinegar
2 tablespoons soy sauce (salt-reduced)
1 clove garlic, finely crushed
1 teaspoon sesame oil
1 teaspoon grated fresh ginger

Combine all ingredients. Refrigerate until ready to serve.
Makes about 3/4 cup

Per 1/4 cup: 118kJ/28Cals/1.6g fat

# Spicy tomato dressing

This is really nice tossed through a pasta salad with some chopped
capsicum, mushrooms and corn kernels.

200ml tomato juice
2 tablespoons lemon juice
1 tablespoon chopped fresh parsley
1 teaspoon Worcestershire sauce
dash Tabasco sauce
1/4 teaspoon dried oregano
1/4 teaspoon dried thyme
pinch ground cayenne
freshly ground black pepper

Combine all ingredients. Refrigerate until ready to use.
Makes about 1 cup

Per 1/4 cup: 63kJ/15Cals/0g fat

## Yoghurt dill sauce

This is lovely with any fish, especially seared Atlantic salmon or char-grilled tuna.

200g non-fat skim milk yoghurt
1/4 cup chopped fresh dill
1 tablespoon cider vinegar
freshly ground black pepper to taste

Combine all ingredients. Refrigerate until ready to serve.
Makes about 1 cup

Per 1/4 cup: 127kJ/30Cals/neg. fat

## Piquant sauce

1/2 cup pineapple juice
1/4 cup sugar
1/4 cup white wine vinegar
1 teaspoon soy sauce (salt-reduced)
1 teaspoon tomato sauce
1/2 tablespoon cornflour

Place all ingredients except cornflour in a small saucepan and stir over gentle heat until boiling. Mix cornflour to a paste with a little water and add to sauce, stirring constantly. Cook until sauce boils and thickens. Good to serve with barbecued beef and pork steaks.
Makes about 1 cup

Per 1/4 cup: 266kJ/63Cals/0g fat

## Tomato sauce

If you have it to hand, add a splash of vodka to give this sauce a delightful kick. It's great served with lean pork kebabs, barbecued steak and chicken.

1/4 cup tomato paste
1/4 cup water
1 tablespoon grated horseradish
2 teaspoons freshly squeezed lemon juice
1 teaspoon Worcestershire sauce
freshly ground black pepper to taste

Combine all ingredients. Will keep in the refrigerator for 2–3 days.
Makes about 3/4 cup

Per 1/4 cup: 120kJ/28Cals/0.3g fat


## Apple and mustard dressing

This is great with a pasta and vegetable salad.

2 tablespoons balsamic vinegar
1 tablespoon apple juice concentrate
1/4 teaspoon French mustard
pinch dried marjoram
salt and freshly ground black pepper to taste

Combine all ingredients and chill well before serving over a pasta salad.
Make about 1/4 cup.

Per 1/4 cup: 85kJ/20Cals/0g fat

# Honey ginger salad dressing

100g non-fat skim milk yoghurt
1 teaspoon honey
1 teaspoon chopped crystallised ginger
1/8 teaspoon ground cumin
pinch cayenne pepper

Combine all ingredients and chill well before serving.
Makes about 1/2 cup

Per 1/4 cup: 210kJ/50Cals/0.1g fat

# Chilli orange dipping sauce

2 tablespoons concentrated orange juice
1 tablespoon chilli sauce
1 tablespoon Worcestershire sauce
1/2 tablespoon lemon juice
1/2 tablespoon sugar
1 small clove garlic, mashed
salt and pepper to taste

Place all ingredients in a lidded jar. Shake well to combine. This
sauce can be stored for up to 1 week if kept in an airtight container
in the refrigerator.
Makes about 1/3 cup

Per 1 tablespoon: 55kJ/13Cals/0g fat

# Coleslaw dressing

This is good with other salads as well, and can also be used as a spread in salad sandwiches. It will keep in an airtight container for 2–3 days in the refrigerator.

1/3 cup thick-style non-fat yoghurt
1/4 cup low-fat buttermilk
1 tablespoon lemon juice
1 teaspoon Worcestershire sauce
few dashes Tabasco sauce
1 teaspoon sugar (optional)
1 teaspoon celery seeds
salt and pepper to taste
1/4 cup chopped fresh parsley

Combine all ingredients. Chill for 30 minutes before serving to allow flavours to blend. Serve tossed through cabbage and carrot slaw.
Makes about 1 cup

Per 1/4 cup: 93kJ/22Cals/0.12g fat

# Roasted yellow capsicum sauce

This is delicious served with seafood, chicken or salads. It will keep in the refrigerator for up to 4 days.

2 yellow capsicums
1 teaspoon white wine vinegar
1 clove garlic, mashed
salt and pepper to taste
1/4 cup thick-style non-fat yoghurt

Grill capsicum until charred all over, about 5–8 minutes. Place in a paper bag for 10 minutes, then remove the skin, core and seeds. Place in a food processor with the vinegar, garlic, salt and pepper. Puree until smooth. Spoon into a bowl and stir in the yoghurt. Refrigerate until ready to serve.
Makes about 1 cup

Per 1/4 cup:111kJ/26Cals/neg fat


# Mango salsa

This is lovely served with seafood, chicken or pork. It will keep in the refrigerator for 2–3 days.

1 large ripe mango, skin and stone removed, flesh chopped
1 small red onion, very finely chopped
1/2 teaspoon very finely chopped chilli (or to taste)
juice 1 lime
2 tablespoons chopped fresh coriander
1/2 tablespoon chopped fresh basil

Combine all ingredients. Cover and refrigerate for at least 30 minutes to allow flavours to blend.
Makes about 1 cup

Per 1/4 cup: 166kJ/39Cals/0g fat

# Spiced tomato jam

This is great to serve with char-grilled steak or chicken. It will keep, refrigerated, for up to 1 week.

750g ripe tomatoes, peeled, seeded and chopped
1 small onion, very finely chopped
1 clove garlic, mashed
1 tablespoon tomato paste
1/2 tablespoon honey
1/4 teaspoon minced ginger
1/2 teaspoon cinnamon
1/4 cup chopped fresh coriander

Place the tomatoes, onion and garlic in a heavy-based frypan over moderate heat. Cook, stirring from time to time, until reduced and thickened. The time will vary depending on the juiciness of the tomatoes but it will probably take about 15 minutes.

Add the tomato paste, honey, ginger and cinnamon and continue cooking until tomatoes reach the consistency of a chutney. Stir through the coriander. Place in a sterilised jar, allow to cool, then refrigerate until ready to serve.
Makes about 2 cups

Per 1/4 cup: 92kJ/22Cals/0g fat

# Balsamic cherry pickle

Really wonderful served with chicken, pork or other cold meats, this pickle will keep refrigerated for up to 1 week.

1 cup balsamic vinegar
125ml water
1/4 cup dark brown sugar
1 strip lemon peel
1 cinnamon stick
5 whole cloves
4 whole allspice berries
2 whole juniper berries
400g ripe cherries, stems removed

Place all ingredients except cherries in a heavy-based stainless steel saucepan. Simmer, uncovered, for 10 minutes or until slightly reduced. Pierce each cherry several times with a needle and place in a sterilised jar. Pour vinegar mixture over to cover the cherries completely. Cover with a clean cloth and allow to cool completely. Seal jar and stand at room temperature for 24 hours before serving. Refrigerate after that.
Makes about 4 cups

Per 1/4 cup: 101kJ/24Cals/0g fat

# Sweet chilli sauce

This sauce will keep for up to a month in the refrigerator—if it's not eaten first!

12 small red chillies, stems removed, finely chopped
2 large cloves garlic, finely chopped
1 cup white wine vinegar
1/2 cup sugar
1 teaspoon salt

Place all the ingredients in a stainless steel saucepan and stir over gentle heat until the sugar has dissolved. Bring to the boil, reduce heat and simmer for 10–15 minutes or until the liquid turns to a syrupy consistency. Pour into warm sterilised jars, then seal.
Makes about 1½ cups

Per tablespoon: 97kJ/23Cals/0g fat


# Port and redcurrant sauce

Serve with chicken, turkey, pork or lamb. This can be used as a sandwich spread for cold meats and salads and will keep for several weeks if stored in a covered, sterilised jar in the refrigerator.

1/3 cup redcurrant jelly
1/4 cup port
grated zest and juice 1 orange
juice 1/2 lemon
1 teaspoon dry mustard powder
1/2 teaspoon grated fresh ginger

Place all ingredients into a small saucepan and heat until thoroughly combined. Pour into a serving dish and allow to go cold before serving.
Makes about 1 cup

Per tablespoon: 148kJ/35Cals/0g fat

# Apple and onion sauce

1 small onion, finely chopped
1/4 cup white wine
2 medium Granny Smith apples, peeled, cored and chopped
2 tablespoons dry cider
1 tablespoon sugar
2 cloves

Simmer the onion in the wine over gentle heat until softened. Add the apples and continue cooking for a further 2 minutes, stirring occasionally, before adding the remaining ingredients. Cover and cook until apples are really soft. Remove the cloves, then puree through a sieve or in a food processor. This sauce is great with pork, ham and lamb.
Makes about 1 cup

Per tablespoon: 91kJ/21Cals/0g fat


# Redcurrant-mint sauce

This is wonderful with lamb and can be used as a spread for lamb sandwiches.

1/3 cup redcurrant jelly
$1\frac{1}{2}$ tablespoons chopped fresh mint
grated rind 1 orange

Combine all ingredients in a bowl.
Makes approx. 1/2 cup

Per tablespoon: 166kJ/39Cals/0g fat

# Mornay sauce

Use this sauce for dishes like lasagna, or pour over vegetables.

2 cups skim milk
1 small carrot, chopped
1 onion, chopped
1 stick celery, chopped
1 clove garlic, crushed
2 cloves
pinch nutmeg
2 tablespoons flour
salt and pepper to taste
1/3 cup grated Parmesan cheese

Simmer the milk, carrot, onion, celery, garlic, cloves and nutmeg for 15–20 minutes. Strain milk and discard the vegetables. Place the flour into a saucepan. Mix a little of the milk into the flour until smooth, then add remaining milk and salt and pepper to taste, and whisk until well combined. Place over gentle heat and cook until sauce boils and thickens. Add the Parmesan cheese and stir until melted and combined.
Makes about 2 cups

Per 1/2 cup: 362kJ/86Cals/2.15g fat

# 17 Snacks

## Salmon dip

210g pink salmon, drained, skin and bones removed
1/2 cup non-fat yoghurt
1 tablespoon snipped chives
dash Tabasco sauce
salt and pepper to taste
assorted vegetable crudités (e.g. carrots, capsicum, celery)

Place salmon in a bowl and flake. Add remaining ingredients and mash together well. Serve with vegetable sticks.
Serves 4

Per serve: 388kJ/92Cals/3.3g fat


## Spicy eggplant garlic dip

1 large eggplant, cut in half lengthwise
1 large clove garlic
1/2 teaspoon chopped fresh chilli
1/2 tablespoon lemon juice
salt and pepper to taste
1/3 cup chopped fresh parsley

Grill eggplant, cut-side down, under a medium hot grill, until the skin is blistered and the flesh is soft. Scoop flesh into a food processor. Add the garlic, chilli, lemon juice, salt and pepper. Process until smooth. Fold through the parsley. Serve with crudités or pita chips (see page 204).
Serves 4

Per serve: 115kJ/27Cals/0g fat

# Pizza-flavoured popcorn

You need a microwave for this recipe to pop the corn without adding any fat. You'll find jars of ready-made herb and spice mix pizza toppings in the herb and spice section of your supermarket under famous brand names.

dried popcorn kernels
herb and spice mix pizza topping

The amount of popcorn prepared in each batch will depend on the size of the container used and the size of your microwave. Simply follow the directions on the popcorn packet. It only takes a few seconds to have beautiful popcorn. While still hot, sprinkle with pizza topping.

Per cup: 115kJ/27Cals/0g fat

# Guilt-free potato chips

2 large Desiree potatoes
pinch salt
malt vinegar to taste

Preheat oven to 180°C. Scrub the potatoes well, but there is no need to peel them. Slice into thin rounds (about 3mm thick). Place directly on oven shelves and bake until crisp, about 10 minutes. The time will depend on the water content of the potatoes. Place in a serving bowl and sprinkle with salt and vinegar.
Serves 2

Per serve: 540kJ/128Cals/0g fat

# Chickpea snack

200g canned chickpeas, drained
1 teaspoon garlic powder
1 teaspoon onion powder
1/2 teaspoon dry mustard powder
1/2 teaspoon turmeric
1/2 teaspoon cracked black pepper
1/4 teaspoon cayenne pepper
1/4 teaspoon chilli powder
1/4 teaspoon roast chicken seasoning salt

Place chickpeas in a bowl. Combine remaining ingredients and sprinkle over chickpeas before serving. The seasoning mix is enough for several batches and can be stored in an airtight jar for 1–2 months.
Serves 4

Per serve: 280kJ/66Cals/1.25g fat

# Spicy crab dip

210g can crab meat, drained
200g non-fat plain yoghurt
1 spring onion, chopped
1/4 teaspoon chilli powder
dash Tabasco sauce
1/4 teaspoon grated fresh ginger
salt and pepper to taste

Combine all ingredients, cover and refrigerate for 1 hour to allow flavours to blend. Serve with crudités, pita chips or toast triangles.
Serves 4

Per serve: 345kJ/82Cals/0.6g fat

# Cottage cheese, pineapple and gherkin dip

1/2 cup low-fat cottage cheese
210g can crushed pineapple, drained
4 small gherkins, chopped
2 tablespoons chopped fresh parsley
salt and pepper to taste

Drain the cottage cheese if necessary, then mix together with the pineapple, gherkins, parsley, salt and pepper. Refrigerate for 1 hour to allow flavours to blend. Serve with crudités or low-fat rice crackers.
Makes about 1½ cups

Per 1/4 cup: 166kJ/39Cals/0.5g fat

# Garlic pita crisps

1 large pita bread
2 large cloves garlic, peeled
pinch salt

Preheat oven to 200°C. With a sharp knife slice around the rim of the pita bread to open it out into two circles. Mash the garlic with the salt to a smooth paste. Spread over both pieces of pita bread, then cut into bite-size pieces. Place on a baking tray and bake in the oven for 8–10 minutes or until crisp.
Serves 4

Per serve: 297kJ/70Cals/0.5g fat

# Mushroom pâté

I use flat mushrooms for this recipe because they have a stronger flavour than cup or button mushrooms and so make a tastier pâté.

4 large flat mushrooms
1 small leek, washed and chopped
1 clove garlic, crushed
1/2 cup beef stock
1 tablespoon dry sherry
cracked black pepper to taste
1/4 cup fine, fresh wholemeal breadcrumbs

Wipe the mushrooms with damp paper towel, then chop. Place the leek and garlic in a saucepan with 1/4 cup beef stock and simmer until softened. Add mushrooms, remaining stock, sherry and pepper. Cover and simmer until mushrooms are cooked. Blend in a food processor until smooth, then place in a bowl and add the breadcrumbs. If the mixture is too runny add more breadcrumbs; if a little too dry, add more sherry or stock. Serve with triangles of toast, pita chips or crudités.
Serves 4

Per serve: 265kJ/63Cals/0g fat

# Cheesy capsicum spread

100g low-fat ricotta cheese
1/2 small red capsicum, finely chopped
1/2 small yellow capsicum, finely chopped
1 stalk celery, finely chopped
1 tablespoon finely chopped fresh parsley
1/2 tablespoon Dijon mustard
15g sultanas, cut in half
salt and pepper to taste
ground paprika

Mash the ricotta in a bowl, then mix through remaining ingredients except paprika. Spoon into a serving dish and sprinkle with paprika. Cover and refrigerate for 1 hour to allow flavour to develop. Serve with toast triangles or low-fat rice crackers.
Serves 4

Per serve: 236kJ/56Cals/2.25g fat


# Salmon and cucumber bites

1 cucumber, cut diagonally into 5mm slices
1/3 cup thick-style non-fat yoghurt
1 tablespoon capers
1 tablespoon snipped chives
100g smoked salmon, cut into bite-size pieces
freshly ground black pepper
dill sprigs

Place the cucumber slices on a flat surface. Spread with combined yoghurt, capers and chives. Top with a piece of salmon, freshly ground black pepper and a sprig of dill and serve immediately.
Serves 6

Per serve: 166kJ/39Cals/0.75g fat

# Three bean dip

300g can three bean mix
1 clove garlic, crushed
2 tablespoons mango chutney
1 tablespoon finely chopped parsley
dash Tabasco sauce
cracked black pepper to taste

Drain the beans and place in a food processor with the garlic. Puree until smooth, place in a bowl and stir through the chutney, parsley, Tabasco and pepper. Place into a serving dish and serve with pita bread or crudités.
Serves 6

Per serve: 303kJ/72Cals/0.25g fat


# Snow peas stuffed with cheese and prawns

12 snow peas, topped and tailed
6 medium cooked prawns, shelled, deveined, chopped
1/2 cup low-fat cottage cheese
1 teaspoon finely chopped coriander
1 teaspoon grated lemon zest
1 teaspoon chilli sauce

Blanch the snow peas in boiling water for 1 minute. Drain and plunge into icy water to stop the cooking process. Split the peas down one side so that they open up like a boat. Combine remaining ingredients and fill snow peas with the mixture.
Makes 4 serves

Per serve: 233kJ/55Cals/1.05g fat

# Sun-dried tomato and basil dip

This dip is made with the sun-dried tomatoes sold loose or in dry packs—not the ones packed in oil. It will keep in a covered sterilised jar in the refrigerator for 2–3 days. It is also wonderful tossed through hot cooked pasta.

100g sun-dried tomatoes
1/2 bunch fresh basil
3 cloves garlic, crushed
salt and pepper to taste

Place the tomatoes in a bowl and cover with boiling water. Leave to soak overnight. Drain, reserving some of the soaking water. Wash the basil and strip the leaves from the stems. Place tomatoes in a food processor with the garlic and basil leaves. Process until smooth. Add a little of the soaking liquid if mixture seems too thick. Scrape into a bowl and season to taste with salt and pepper. Serve with crudités and/or low-fat rice crackers.
Makes about 1½ cups

Per 1/4 cup: 160kJ/38Cals/0g fat

# Cheese and herb morsels

2 slices lavash bread
1 cup low-fat cottage cheese
1 Lebanese cucumber, peeled, seeded and finely chopped
1 teaspoon grated lemon zest
1/2 tablespoon chopped fresh mint
1/2 tablespoon chopped fresh basil
1/2 tablespoon chopped fresh parsley
1/2 tablespoon snipped chives
salt and pepper to taste

Place the bread on a flat surface. Combine remaining ingredients and spread over bread. Roll up and cut into bite-size pieces, securing bread with toothpicks.
Makes about 16 morsels

Per morsel: 150kJ/35Cals/0.5g fat


# Sweet potato and pumpkin crisps

250g sweet potato, peeled
250g pumpkin, peeled

Preheat oven to 180°C. Thinly slice both sweet potato and pumpkin. Place in one layer on a large non-stick baking sheet or tray lined with non-stick baking paper. Bake for 30–45 minutes until crisp (time will vary depending on the moisture content of the vegetables), turning over halfway through cooking time. Remove from oven and allow to cool on a wire rack.
Serves 4

Per serve: 275kJ/65Cals/0g fat

# Crab, cheese and cucumber cups

4 slices wholemeal bread, crusts removed
1 cup low-fat cottage cheese
1/2 cup crab meat, drained
1 Lebanese cucumber, peeled, seeded and finely chopped
1 tablespoon chilli sauce
dash Tabasco sauce
salt and pepper to taste

Preheat oven to 150°C. Spray bread slices with a little water and press into small muffin cups. Bake for 15–20 minutes or until crunchy. Meanwhile combine remaining ingredients. Remove bread cups from oven and allow to cool. Fill with crab mixture and serve.
Makes 4

Per serve: 615kJ/146Cals/2.75g fat

# Spicy tomato dip

4 ripe tomatoes, peeled, seeded and finely chopped
4 spring onions, finely chopped
1 tablespoon lemon juice
1 tablespoon chopped fresh coriander
1 teaspoon chopped fresh chilli
salt and pepper to taste

Combine all ingredients in a bowl. Cover and refrigerate for 1 hour to allow flavours to blend. Serve with pita chips or crudités.
Serves 4

Per serve: 115kJ/27Cals/0g fat

# 18 Desserts

## Almond, date and rice pudding

Even though this dessert takes one and half hours to cook, you only have to spend about 5 minutes preparing it, so you can go off and do other things while it's baking. It's wonderful comfort food and tastes wicked, even though it's not.

1/4 cup short grain rice
30g dried dates, chopped
15g flaked almonds
1½ cups low-fat milk
1/2 tablespoon honey
1/4 teaspoon almond or vanilla essence
1/8 teaspoon ground cardamom

Preheat oven to 180°C. Place the rice, dates and almonds in a small casserole dish. Combine the milk, honey, essence and cardamom in a saucepan and bring to the boil, stirring constantly, then pour over rice. Bake uncovered for 1 hour, then cover with foil and continue cooking for a further 30 minutes.
Serves 2

Per serve: 1352kJ/322Cals/6.6g fat

# Crunchy baked apples

1 tablespoon caster sugar
1 tablespoon soft brown sugar
1 tablespoon finely chopped walnuts
1 teaspoon ground cinnamon
2 Granny Smith apples, peeled and cored
2 tablespoons apricot jam, melted

Preheat oven to 180°C. Combine sugars, walnuts and cinnamon. Place apples in a baking dish, brush with melted jam. Press walnut mixture onto apples. Bake for about 30 minutes or until apples are tender. This is nice served with Low-fat Butterscotch Sauce (p. 213). Serves 2

Per serve: 839kJ/199Cals/2g fat

# Vanilla topping

This goes well with just about any pudding from apple crumble to pancakes—anywhere you'd use a dollop of whipped cream, in fact.

1/2 cup non-fat cottage cheese
1/2 cup non-fat plain yoghurt
2 tablespoons honey
1/4 teaspoon vanilla essence

Combine all ingredients. Cover and refrigerate. This will keep in the refrigerator until the earlier use-by date on the yoghurt or cottage cheese.
Makes about 1/2 cups

Per tablespoon: 269kJ/64Cals/0.5g fat

# Low-fat butterscotch sauce

This sauce makes more than you need for two servings, but making it in smaller quantities is not practical. It will keep in the refrigerator for 2–3 days. Serve it with canned or stewed fruit for another dessert.

1 tablespoon dark brown sugar
1 tablespoon golden syrup
$1\frac{1}{2}$ cups skim milk
1 small egg
2 tablespoons cornflour
1/2 teaspoon vanilla essence

Combine the sugar and syrup in a small saucepan over low heat, stirring until sugar dissolves. Simmer for 1 minute. Slowly stir in 3/4 cup milk and heat until hot but not boiling. Beat the egg, then stir in the remaining milk, cornflour and vanilla essence. Add to pan, stirring constantly until sauce boils and thickens.
Makes about 2 cups

Per 1/4 cup: 225kJ/53Cals/0.73g fat

# Sultana, ginger and ricotta pastries

1/4 cup low-fat ricotta cheese
2 tablespoons thick-style non-fat yoghurt
2 tablespoons sultanas
2 tablespoons chopped glace ginger
1 teaspoon grated lemon zest
1 teaspoon brown sugar
2 sheets filo pastry
1/4 cup skim milk
1 tablespoon runny honey
caster sugar

Preheat oven to 200°C. Combine cheese, yoghurt, sultanas, ginger, lemon and sugar. Combine milk and honey. Working with one sheet of filo at a time, brush with milk mixture and fold in half. Brush again with milk mixture and place half the ricotta mixture into the centre of the pastry, then fold up into a parcel, brushing with milk mixture at each fold. Place on a non-stick baking sheet, seam-side down. Brush again with milk mixture and sprinkle with caster sugar. Bake for 5–10 minutes or until crisp and golden. Serve with non-fat yoghurt which has been sweetened with a little honey, if liked.
Serves 2

Per serve: 1005kJ/239Cals/4.1g fat

# Spiced fruit compote

1/4 cup chopped dates
1/4 cup pitted prunes
1/4 cup chopped dried pears
1/4 cup dried apricots
300ml apple juice
1/2 cinnamon stick
1/4 teaspoon mixed spice
1 clove
1 tablespoon brandy

Place the fruit in a bowl and pour over apple juice, then add the cinnamon stick, mixed spice and clove. Stir well. Cover and macerate overnight.

Place fruit and liquid in a saucepan and simmer for 20 minutes. Remove from heat and stir in the brandy. Serve hot or cold with non-fat plain yoghurt sweetened with a little honey.
Serves 2

Per serve: 1270kJ/302Cals/ 0g fat

# Figs poached in red wine

1 cup red wine
2 tablespoons caster sugar
2 tablespoons orange juice
2 tablespoons lemon juice
1 tablespoon blackcurrant liqueur (optional)
4 fresh figs
1/4 cup non-fat yoghurt
orange shreds for decoration

Place the red wine, sugar, orange juice, lemon juice and liqueur in a stainless steel or glass saucepan. Stir over gentle heat until sugar dissolves. Add the figs and simmer gently for 5 minutes, basting the figs with the liquid from time to time. Remove to a serving dish with a slotted spoon. Increase heat and simmer liquid, stirring constantly, until sauce thickens slightly. Pour over figs. They can be served warm, or chilled in the poaching sauce and served cold. Serve with a spoonful of yoghurt decorated with orange shreds.
Serves 2

Per serve: 1141kJ/271Cals/0g fat

# Pear and ginger self-saucing pudding

My good friend Maree Peden, from 'Bullamalita' on the Southern Tablelands of New South Wales, gave me this recipe, which she makes using apples. As I was replacing the butter in the original recipe with apple sauce I felt pears would work well—and they do. I have also used the sugar substitute Splenda™ to cut down on the kilojoules. It's surprisingly simple and absolutely delicious.

2 pears, peeled, cored and chopped
2 tablespoons sultanas
1 teaspoon grated fresh ginger
1 teaspoon grated lemon rind
3/4 cup self-raising flour, sifted
1/2 cup Splenda™
1/4 cup apple puree
1 egg white
2 tablespoons cold water (approx.)
2 tablespoons brown sugar
2 tablespoons hot water

Preheat the oven to 180°C. Place pears in a non-stick ovenproof dish (see note) and sprinkle evenly with sultanas, ginger and lemon rind. Sift flour and Splenda™ into a bowl, make a well in the centre, add apple puree, egg white and enough cold water to make a cake-like batter. Beat with a wooden spoon until smooth. Spread mixture over pears. Sift brown sugar evenly over top of pudding, gently pour hot water over the sugar. Bake uncovered for 50–60 minutes or until cooked when tested. Serve with a dollop of non-fat yoghurt sweetened with a little honey, if liked.

*Note:* The uncooked pears and topping should fill the dish by no more than two-thirds, so use a dish big enough to accommodate this. If the dish is overfilled the pudding will spill over the sides as it rises and you will lose all the lovely sauce.

Serves 2

Per serve:1680kJ/400Cals/0.5g fat

# Apple snow

A dessert from my childhood but still great!

1 large Granny Smith apple, peeled, cored and chopped
2 tablespoons water
1 tablespoon caster sugar
pinch nutmeg (or to taste)
2 egg whites
1 tablespoon caster sugar, extra

Simmer the apple in a small saucepan with the water and sugar until tender. Cool slightly, then puree in a food processor or push through a fine sieve. Allow to cool completely, then stir through a pinch of nutmeg.

Beat egg whites and sugar in a clean dry bowl until stiff and glossy. Fold one spoonful of egg white through the apple, then fold through remaining egg white. Spoon into serving dishes and chill.
Serves 2

Per serve: 500kJ/119Cals/0g fat

# Strawberries with meringue topping

1 small punnet strawberries, washed and hulled
2 tablespoons apple juice
1 tablespoon strawberry liqueur
1 egg white
2 tablespoons caster sugar
1/2 tablespoon icing sugar
2 tablespoons brown sugar

Place strawberries in a bowl. Combine the apple juice and strawberry liqueur and pour over strawberries. Cover and macerate overnight. Drain strawberries and reserve marinade. Spoon strawberries into 2 heatproof ramekins.

Preheat oven to 160°C. Beat egg white until stiff. Gradually add the sugar and continue to beat until stiff and glossy. Spoon over the strawberries. Dust with sifted icing sugar. Bake for 10–15 minutes or until meringue starts to turn golden brown.

Meanwhile, place reserved marinade and brown sugar in a small saucepan and simmer over medium heat until reduced and thickened slightly. Spoon onto two serving plates, then spoon meringue and strawberries over.
Serves 2

Per serve: 746kJ/177Cals/0g fat

# Caramel grapes with vanilla yoghurt

200g non-fat plain yoghurt
1 teaspoon honey
1/4 teaspoon vanilla essence (or to taste)
125g seedless grapes, washed and halved
1/3 cup sugar

Combine the yoghurt, honey and vanilla and spoon into two ramekin dishes. Top with grapes. Place the sugar in a small saucepan, add just enough water to cover it and stir until completely dissolved. Then boil over high heat until dark golden brown. Pour over grapes and serve.
Serves 2

Per serve: 1025kJ/244Cals/0.25g fat


# Caramel oranges

1 large navel orange, cut in half
2 tablespoons Grand Marnier
2 tablespoons dark brown sugar

Cut a slice from each end of orange so that the halves stand level when placed cut-side up. Cut segments loose from the pith but leave in place. Sprinkle each half with Grand Marnier, then sprinkle on the brown sugar. Place oranges under hot grill and cook until sugar has melted and become bubbly. Serve with a dollop of non-fat yoghurt sweetened with a little honey.
Serves 2

Per serve: 579kJ/137Cals/0g fat

# Ricotta with raspberry coulis

1/2 cup low-fat ricotta cheese
1/4 cup non-fat plain yoghurt
1 teaspoon vanilla essence
1 egg white
1½ tablespoons icing sugar
1 small punnet raspberries
1½ tablespoons caster sugar (or to taste)
1 tablespoon raspberry liqueur
mint sprigs (optional)

Combine the ricotta, yoghurt and vanilla until smooth. Beat the egg white until stiff peaks begin to form, then sift in the icing sugar. Fold one spoonful of egg white mixture into the ricotta mixture, then carefully fold through remaining egg white until well combined. Place into two dampened ramekins, cover and refrigerate until required.

Meanwhile puree the raspberries, then pass through a fine sieve. Place in a bowl with the sugar and liqueur and stir until the sugar dissolves. Cover and refrigerate until required.

To serve, unmould ricotta onto a serving plate, spoon raspberry coulis around it, and decorate with a mint sprig.
Serves 2

Per serve: 1004kJ/239Cals/7g fat

# Summer pudding

12 slices white bread, crusts removed
500g mixed berries (e.g. strawberries, raspberries, blueberries, blackberries)
1/3 cup caster sugar
1 tablespoon lemon juice
1 tablespoon strawberry or raspberry liqueur

Cut 1 slice of bread into a circle the diameter of the slice. Cut the rest of the bread slices into fingers about 3cm wide. Place the circle of bread in the base of a 3-cup capacity bowl. Line the rest of the bowl with bread fingers, overlapping them as you go and reserving enough bread to cover the top.

Place the berries in a saucepan with the sugar, lemon juice and liqueur and simmer gently for 5 minutes. Remove from the heat. Spoon some of the syrup over the bread in the base of the bowl, then spoon berries into the bowl with a slotted spoon. Cover the top of the bowl with the remaining bread so there are no gaps. Brush with the syrup; retain remaining syrup. Place a piece of foil over the pudding, then a small plate that fits just on top of the pudding. Place a heavy weight (like a can of beans) on the plate and refrigerate overnight.

Remove weight and foil from bowl and unmould onto a serving plate. Brush with remaining syrup and serve decorated with a sprig of mint.
Serves 4

Per serve: 641kJ/152Cals/2.1g fat

# Strawberry delight

1 small punnet strawberries, washed and hulled
1 tablespoon boiling water
1 teaspoon gelatine
1 teaspoon caster sugar
200g non-fat plain yoghurt
1 egg white
1 tablespoon caster sugar, extra

Place strawberries in a food processor. Combine the boiling water and gelatine and stir until smooth, then add to strawberries with the sugar. Process until smooth. Strain into a bowl and stir through the yoghurt. Whip the egg white until peaks form. Sift in the extra sugar and continue beating until stiff and glossy. Fold 1 spoonful of egg white through yoghurt mixture, then fold through the remainder. Place in serving bowls and chill before serving.
Serves 4

Per serve: 247kJ/58Cals/0.1g fat

# Apple and blackberry crumble

2 Granny Smith apples, peeled, cored and chopped
1 small punnet blackberries
1/2 cup caster sugar
1 cup 1-minute oats
1/2 cup wholemeal self-raising flour
1/3 cup apple sauce

Preheat oven to 180°C. Arrange the apples and blackberries in a baking dish. Sprinkle with 1 tablespoon sugar. Spoon over 2 tablespoons water. Combine remaining ingredients and spoon over the top. Bake for 20–25 minutes or until golden brown on top.
Serves 4

Per serve: 1334kJ/317Cals/0.37g fat

# Fruit salad with sherried yoghurt

100ml non-fat plain yoghurt
1 tablespoon sweet sherry
1/4 teaspoon vanilla essence
2 cups mixed fruit salad (strawberries, melon, grapes, oranges, etc.)
1 cup champagne

Combine the yoghurt, sherry and vanilla in a bowl, beat until smooth. Refrigerate until ready to use. Spoon fruit into two serving dishes and pour champagne over. Serve with a dollop of sherried yoghurt.
Serves 2

Per serve: 1093kJ/260Cals/0.1g fat

# Fruit-topped pavlova

4 egg whites
3/4 cup castor sugar
1 teaspoon white wine vinegar
1/2 teaspoon vanilla essence
2 cups mixed fruit (strawberries, kiwifruit, bananas, passionfruit, etc.)
300ml non-fat plain yoghurt
1/4 cup honey

Preheat oven to 150°C. In a clean dry bowl, beat egg whites until soft peaks form. Gradually add the sugar and continue beating until whites are thick and glossy. Fold in vinegar and vanilla. Line a baking sheet with non-stick baking paper. Spoon meringue onto sheet to form a circle. Bake for 30 minutes, then reduce heat to 120°C and continue baking for a further 45 minutes. Switch off heat and leave pavlova to dry out and cool in the oven with the door slightly ajar. Top with fruit and serve with combined yoghurt and honey.
Serves 6

Per serve: 818kJ/194Cals/0.1g fat

# Pear and cinnamon parcels

1 large firm pear, peeled, cored and chopped
1/4 cup sultanas
2 tablespoons water
1/4 teaspoon ground cinnamon
1 clove
pinch cardamom
2 tablespoons skim milk
1 tablespoon liquid honey
2 sheets filo pastry
caster sugar

Cook the pear, sultanas, water, cinnamon, clove and cardamom in a saucepan over gentle heat until pear is tender. Combine the skim milk and honey.

Preheat oven to 200°C. Working with one sheet of filo at a time, brush with milk and honey mixture and fold in half. Brush again with milk mixture and place half of the pear mixture into the centre of the pastry, then fold up into a parcel, brushing with milk mixture at each fold. Place on a non-stick baking sheet, seam-side down. Brush again with milk mixture and sprinkle with caster sugar. Bake for 5–10 minutes or until crisp and golden. Serve with non-fat yoghurt which has been sweetened with a little honey, if liked.
Serves 2

Per serve: 815kJ/194Cals/0.6g fat

# Crunchy pear cobbler

1 cup rolled oats
1/2 cup wholemeal self-raising flour, sifted
1/3 cup brown sugar
1/2 teaspoon ground cinnamon
1 cup apple juice
2 large pears, peeled, cored and chopped

Preheat oven to 180°C. Combine oats, flour, brown sugar and cinnamon. Mix in the apple juice. Spoon a third of the mixture into the base of a 20cm springform pan. Arrange the pears over the top, spoon over remaining oat mixture. Bake for 20–25 minutes or until golden brown.
Serves 4

Per serve: 1117kJ/266Cals/3.4g fat

# Vanilla custard

1/4 cup custard powder
1 tablespoon sugar
1/3 cup skim milk powder
2 cups hot water
2 teaspoons vanilla essence

Combine the custard powder, sugar and milk powder in a saucepan. Gradually stir in the water until mixture is smooth. Bring slowly to the boil over medium heat, stirring constantly. Cook until thickened. Remove from heat and stir in vanilla. Serve with stewed or poached fruit.
Makes about $2\frac{1}{2}$ cups

Per 1/4 cup: 116kJ/27Cals/neg fat

# 19  Baked treats

## Low-fat walnut brownies

These aren't as fudge-like as traditional brownies but they disappear just as fast! A 180g jar of pureed prunes baby food is ideal for this recipe, otherwise soak pitted prunes for an hour or so, then puree in a food processor.

1/2 cup self-raising flour, sifted
2/3 cup caster sugar
1/3 cup cocoa powder
pinch of salt
1/4 cup roughly chopped walnuts
1/2 cup pureed prunes
1 egg
1 egg white
1 teaspoon vanilla essence

Preheat oven to 180°C. Sift the flour, sugar, cocoa and salt into a bowl, then stir through the walnuts. In a separate bowl combine the prunes, egg, egg white and vanilla essence. Stir the prune mixture through the flour mixture until combined. Spoon mixture into a 20cm (8") square non-stick cake tin and bake for 20–25 minutes or until a skewer inserted into the centre comes out clean. Allow to cool, then cut into 5cm (2") squares.
Makes about 25 squares

Per square: 232kJ/55Cals/2g fat

# Lancashire parkin

My mother-in-law Alice Gore was Lancashire born and bred, and baking was an everyday occurrence in her household. This was one of my favourites. I've modified it, but it still tastes great even without the lashings of butter it used to be served with.

$1\frac{1}{2}$ cups oatmeal
$1\frac{1}{2}$ cups self-raising flour
1 teaspoon ground ginger
1/2 teaspoon salt (optional)
1/2 cup brown sugar
1/3 cup black treacle
1/3 cup golden syrup
1/2 cup skim milk
1/2 cup apple puree
1 egg white, lightly beaten

Preheat the oven to 180°C. Line a 22cm square cake tin with non-stick baking paper. Combine the oatmeal, flour, ginger and salt in a large bowl, make a well in the centre.

Place the sugar, treacle, golden syrup and milk in a saucepan and stir over gentle heat until sugar has dissolved and mixture is well combined. Remove from heat and cool slightly.

Combine the apple puree and egg white and mix into the flour, then slowly pour in the treacle mixture, stirring constantly, to make a soft cake batter. You may have to add a little more milk, depending on the flour used. Pour batter into prepared tin and smooth the top. Bake for 40–50 minutes or until top springs back when lightly pressed with a fingertip.

Allow parkin to cool in the tin until just warm before turning out and cooling completely on a wire rack. Cut into squares.
Makes about 20 squares

Per square: 507kJ/120Cals/1g fat

# Quick beer damper

The beer has to be at room temperature for this recipe so don't use a can straight from the refrigerator.

3 cups wholemeal self-raising flour
1/2 tablespoon caster sugar
1 teaspoon salt (optional)
375ml can beer
skim milk
plain white flour

Preheat oven to 220°C. Sift the flour, sugar and salt into a bowl and return any husks to the flour. Using a butter knife, mix in the beer to form a soft dough. With floured hands form into a round and place on a non-stick baking tray (or a tray lined with non-stick baking paper). Score a cross in the top of the dough, brush with skim milk and dust with flour. Bake for 35–40 minutes or until the damper sounds hollow when tapped on its base.
Makes 1 damper (10 slices)

Per slice: 606kJ/144Cals/1g fat

---

- When kneading scone or bread dough don't add too much extra flour as this will be incorporated into the dough and make the scones or bread tough.

---

# Banana pecan fudge squares

2/3 cup 1-minute oats
1 small banana, mashed
1/4 cup roughly chopped pecan nuts
1/2 cup sugar
1/3 cup cocoa powder
1 tablespoon flour
1/4 teaspoon salt (optional)
1/4 cup honey
2 egg whites
1 teaspoon vanilla extract

Preheat oven to 160°C. Combine all ingredients in a large bowl and mix well. Allow to stand for 5 minutes. Meanwhile, line a 20cm square slab tin with non-stick baking paper. Spread mixture evenly into tin and bake for 20–25 minutes, until the centre is just set and the edges are starting to pull away from the sides. Cool in tin, then cut into squares.
Makes about 16 squares

Per square: 355kJ/84Cals/2g fat

# Pumpkin bread

3/4 cup grated pumpkin
1/4 cup freshly grated Parmesan cheese
2 cloves garlic, mashed
1 teaspoon cracked black pepper
1 teaspoon chopped fresh oregano (or 1/4 teaspoon dried oregano)
1 teaspoon dried thyme
3 cups self-raising flour
2 teaspoons sugar
1 teaspoon salt (optional)
30g pumpkin seeds
1½ cups beer at room temperature (not straight from the fridge)

Preheat oven to 200°C. In a large bowl combine the pumpkin, Parmesan, garlic and seasonings. Sift in the flour, sugar and salt. Mix well, then stir through the pumpkin seeds so they are evenly distributed. Stir in enough beer to make a moist dough.

Place in a non-stick 1kg loaf tin and bake for 10 minutes. Reduce heat to 180°C and baking for a further 35 minutes or until the bread is golden brown on the outside and gives a hollow sound when tapped on its base. Cool in the tin for 10 minutes before turning out onto a wire rack to cool completely.

Makes 1 loaf (about 20 slices)

Per slice: 385kJ/91Cals/0.8g fat

# Banana honey drop scones

1 cup self-raising flour
1/4 teaspoon cinnamon
1/4 cup oatmeal
300ml (1¼ cups) skim milk
2 egg whites
2 tablespoons honey
1 tablespoon apple sauce
1/2 cup mashed ripe banana

Sift the flour and cinnamon into a bowl. Stir through the oatmeal. Combine the skim milk, egg whites, honey, apple sauce and mashed banana. Combine with dry ingredients to make a dropping batter. Mix well. Heat a large, non-stick frying pan over medium heat. Drop tablespoons of mixture into hot pan. When bubbles rise to the surface, turn over to cook the other side. Remove from pan when golden brown on both sides. Serve with extra honey and a dollop of non-fat yoghurt, if liked.
Makes about 16

Per scone: 283kJ/67Cals/0.4g fat

# Quick corn bread

2 cups cornmeal (polenta)
2 teaspoons sugar
2 teaspoons baking powder
1 teaspoon salt
1¼ cups skim milk
1 egg, lightly beaten
1 teaspoon olive oil

Preheat oven to 180°C. Place the cornmeal, sugar, baking powder and salt in a bowl and make a well in the centre. Combine remaining ingredients and stir into the cornmeal. Mix well to combine. Spoon into a shallow, non-stick loaf tin. Bake for 25–30 minutes or until a skewer inserted in the centre comes out clean.
Makes 1 loaf (12 slices)

Per slice: 493kJ/117Cals/1.5g fat

---

- Never fill cake, loaf or muffin tins more than two-thirds full. Any more and they will overflow.

---

# Simple date and pecan loaf

180g pitted dates
300ml water
1 cup wholemeal self-raising flour
30g pecans, chopped
1/2 teaspoon vanilla essence
skim milk

Place the dates and water into a saucepan and simmer, stirring occasionally, until dates are soft. Beat until smooth with a wooden spoon.

Preheat oven to 180°C. Sift flour into a bowl, returning the husks to the flour. Stir in the pecans and make a well in the centre. Add the dates and vanilla, adding a little skim milk if mixture seems too dry. Spoon into a non-stick loaf tin. Bake for 50–60 minutes or until a skewer inserted into the centre comes out clean.
Makes 1 loaf (12 slices)

Per slice: 457kJ/108Cals/2g fat

---

- If you like you can use wholemeal flour in place of white flour in most recipes. However, the texture won't be as light. Alternatively, you could use half white flour and half wholemeal flour.

# Apple and walnut scone loaf

2 cups self-raising flour
1/4 cup caster sugar
1 teaspoon ground cinnamon
1 small Granny Smith apple, peeled and grated
1/4 cup walnuts, chopped
1/2 cup low-fat buttermilk
1/2 cup skim milk
2 tablespoons apple sauce
skim milk, extra
cinnamon sugar

Preheat oven to 210°C. Line a baking slide with non-stick baking paper.

Sift the flour, sugar and cinnamon into a bowl. Stir through the apple and walnuts. Make a well in the centre. Combine the buttermilk, skim milk and apple sauce. Pour into flour and mix to a dough, which should be quite sticky. With floured hands pat dough into a round and place on baking slide. Brush with extra milk and sprinkle with cinnamon sugar. Bake for 15–20 minutes or until a skewer inserted into the centre of the loaf comes out clean. Cool on a wire rack. Cut into 12 wedges and serve with jam of choice.
Serves 12

Per wedge: 665kJ/158Cals/1.7g fat

# Date, walnut and banana bread

2 cups wholemeal self-raising flour
1/3 cup brown sugar
90g dried dates, chopped
1/4 cup walnuts, finely chopped
1 egg
1 egg white
1 large banana
1/2 teaspoon vanilla essence
skim milk

Preheat oven to 180°C. Sift the flour into a bowl, returning any husks to the flour afterwards. Stir in the sugar, dates and walnuts. Make a well in the centre. Lightly beat the egg and egg white and stir in well mashed banana and vanilla. Add egg mixture to flour, adding a little skim milk if mixture seems too dry. Spoon mixture into a non-stick loaf tin. Bake for 1 hour or until a skewer inserted in the middle comes out clean. Cool in tin for a few minutes before turning out onto a wire rack to cool completely. Serve with jam of choice.
Makes 1 loaf (12 slices)

Per slice: 604kJ/143Cals/2g fat

> • Allow cakes to stand in the tin for a few minutes before turning out, so they will come away cleanly, without sticking to the tin.

# Mixed fruit tea bread

2 cups dried mixed fruit (sultanas, raisins, currants, dates, etc.)
1 cup soft brown sugar
1 cup black tea
1½ cups wholemeal self-raising flour
1 teaspoon mixed spice
1/2 teaspoon cinnamon
1 egg, beaten
100g glace cherries, chopped

Place the mixed fruit, sugar and tea in a bowl. Cover and allow to macerate overnight.

Preheat oven to 160°C. Sift the flour and spices into a bowl, returning any husks to the flour. Add the egg, glace cherries and fruit and tea mixture, and mix well. Spoon into a non-stick loaf tin and bake for 1 hour or until a skewer inserted into the centre of the loaf comes out clean. Cool in tin for a few minutes before turning out to cool completely on a wire rack. Serve with jam of choice.
Makes 1 loaf (12 slices)

Per slice: 697kJ/166Cals/0.8g fat

> - A cake is cooked if a skewer inserted into the centre comes out clean; if it is a light-textured cake such as a sponge, the top will spring back when pressed lightly with a fingertip.

# 20 Entertaining

Most of the recipes in this section are in quantities to feed four or six people.

## Salmon ramekins with soy ginger dressing

I love raw salmon, but if it doesn't appeal to you, lightly poach or microwave it, then allow it to cool before continuing with the recipe.

8 slices smoked salmon
400g fresh sashimi salmon, all bones removed
2 tablespoons salmon eggs
4 tablespoons light soy sauce (salt-reduced)
2 tablespoons sake or dry sherry
2 tablespoons mirin
1 teaspoon finely chopped ginger
1 tablespoon wasabi paste (optional)
chicory leaves for garnish (optional)
thin lemon wedges

Line 4 small ramekins with smoked salmon, leaving enough hanging over the edges to fold across top. Finely dice salmon fillet and half fill each ramekin. Place half a tablespoon of salmon eggs in each one. Top with remaining salmon. Fold overhanging smoked salmon over top. Cover with plastic wrap and chill well.

Remove plastic wrap and invert ramekins onto serving plates. Shake slightly so that salmon parcel drops gently onto the plate.

Combine the soy sauce, sake or dry sherry, mirin and ginger and pour around the salmon parcels. Garnish with wasabi, chicory and lemon wedges.
Serves 4

Per serve: 860kJ/204Cals/8.5g fat

# Polynesian salmon and tomato salad

360g fresh salmon fillet, all bones removed
1/3 cup lime juice
1 teaspoon sugar
1/2 teaspoon salt, or to taste
2 large ripe tomatoes, peeled, seeded and diced
1/2 teaspoon chopped chilli
2 spring onions, finely chopped
freshly ground pepper to taste
lime wedges and coriander sprigs for garnish

Cut salmon into bite-size slices across the grain and place in a shallow dish. Combine the lime juice, sugar and salt and pour over salmon slices, making sure they are well coated. Cover and refrigerate for at least 4 hours or overnight, turning occasionally. Drain salmon. Combine tomatoes, chilli and onions and season to taste with pepper. Pour tomato mixture over salmon and toss gently together. Place on serving plates and garnish with lime wedges and coriander sprigs.
Serves 2

Per serve: 1097kJ/261Cals/10.8g fat

# Seafood pasta

This is really quick and easy for entertaining as you can make the sauce the day before and store it, covered, in the refrigerator. Then all you have to do is cook the pasta and heat the seafood in the sauce, which only takes 3–5 minutes.

1 medium onion, peeled and chopped
1 clove garlic, crushed
1/2 cup chicken stock
2 large ripe tomatoes, peeled, seeded and chopped
4 anchovy fillets, drained on paper towel, mashed
1 tablespoon Worcestershire sauce
1/2 teaspoon dried mixed herbs
1/4 teaspoon chopped chilli
dash Tabasco sauce
12 green king prawns, peeled and deveined
1 calamari hood, cut into bite-sized pieces and scored in a
diamond pattern on one side
400g ling fillet, cut into large bite-sized pieces
4 cups hot cooked pasta
chopped parsley

Sweat the onion and garlic in the stock until tender, about 3 minutes. Add the tomatoes, anchovy fillets, Worcestershire sauce, herbs, chilli and Tabasco sauce. Simmer, stirring occasionally, until sauce thickens, about 10–15 minutes. At this point the sauce can be cooled, and refrigerated until next day.

Have the seafood prepared and ready. Cook pasta and bring sauce to the simmer in another saucepan. Three to four minutes before the pasta is ready add the seafood to the tomato sauce and cook, stirring occasionally, until the prawns and fish turn opaque. Don't overcook. Serve pasta with seafood sauce sprinkled with chopped parsley.
Serves 4

Per serve: 1515kJ/360Cals/3.35g fat

# Grilled Atlantic salmon with fennel and walnuts

4 Atlantic salmon steaks (about 180g each)
1 small bulb fennel, washed and sliced
1/2 cup dry vermouth
1 clove garlic, crushed
1/4 cup chopped fresh parsley
salt and pepper to taste

Place the salmon steaks in a shallow dish and arrange fennel slices over the top. Combine remaining ingredients and pour over salmon. Cover and marinate for 30 minutes. Remove salmon steaks from marinade and place on a foil-lined grill tray. Place fennel and marinade in a saucepan and gently simmer until fennel is tender, about 10 minutes.

Meanwhile, heat grill to medium hot and grill salmon for 5 minutes on each side or until cooked to taste. Serve salmon with fennel, plain boiled potatoes and a salad of mixed greens with rocket, watercress and radicchio.
Serves 4

Per serve: 762kJ/181Cals/7g fat

# Braised ocean salmon

1kg saddle ocean salmon
1½ cups fish or vegetable stock
1 large onion, chopped
2 cloves garlic, crushed
1 stalk celery, chopped
1/2 cup chopped parsley
1 cup white wine
425g can peeled tomatoes, chopped
1/4 cup tomato paste
2 bay leaves
salt and pepper to taste

Ask your fish shop to remove any scales from the salmon. Wash thoroughly and pat dry. In a heavy-based saucepan large enough to hold the salmon, place 1/2 cup stock, onion, garlic and celery and simmer gently until softened. Add the remaining stock, parsley, wine, tomatoes, tomato paste, bay leaves and seasoning. Simmer for 10 minutes. Add salmon to the pan and baste with the sauce. Cover and simmer for 20 minutes.

Check the fish to see if it is cooked through—it will depend on how thick the saddle is—then continue cooking until flesh flakes easily with a fork. Serve with pan juices, plain boiled potatoes and lemon wedges.
Serves 6

Per serve: 893kJ/212gCals/7g fat

# Bouillabaisse

I use the prawn shells and fish trimmings, if any, to make a fish stock (see page 131) for this dish. The stock only takes 20 minutes to simmer while I am preparing all the other ingredients. At a pinch you can use chicken stock but it doesn't give the same rich flavour as fish stock does. With all the ingredients prepared ready to use, bouillabaisse takes very little time to cook before serving. You'll need a really large saucepan and serving tureen.

1 large leek, washed well and chopped
2 cloves garlic, crushed
1½ cups white wine
3 large ripe tomatoes, peeled, seeded and chopped
10cm strip orange peel
1 bouquet garni
1 sprig fresh fennel leaves
3 cups fish stock
1/4 teaspoon ground nutmeg
1/4 teaspoon ground saffron
salt and pepper to taste
500g ling fillet, cut into large bite-size pieces
12 green king prawns, peeled (tails left intact), deveined
12 scallops
12 mussels, well scrubbed and debearded
3 cooked blue swimmer crabs, halved and cleaned
2 tablespoons chopped parsley

In a large, heavy-based saucepan, simmer the leek, garlic and 1/2 cup white wine until leek has softened. Add the tomatoes, orange peel, bouquet garni, fennel, fish stock, nutmeg, saffron and remaining wine. Bring to the boil, reduce heat and simmer, skimming away any scum that rises to the surface, for 5 minutes. Taste and season with salt and pepper.

Add the ling and simmer for 3 minutes, add the prawns and

continue cooking for a further 2 minutes, add remaining ingredients and continue cooking until scallops become opaque, mussels open and crab warms through, about a further 3 minutes.

Remove the bouquet garni, fennel sprigs and orange peel. Ladle into a large, warmed tureen or serving bowl, sprinkle with chopped parsley and serve with plenty of crusty bread to mop up the broth. Serves 6

Per serve: 1280kJ/304Cals/3.4g fat

# Rainbow trout with orange and ginger

4 rainbow trout, cleaned and prepared
12 slices fresh ginger root
1 teaspoon grated fresh ginger
1/2 cup orange juice
2 tablespoons brown sugar

Cut three diagonal slashes on each side of the trout to prevent them curling up during cooking. Place three slices of ginger in the cavity of each fish. Line a grill tray with foil and place the fish on it.

Preheat grill to medium high. Place grated ginger, orange juice and brown sugar in a small saucepan, bring to the boil, stirring until all the sugar has dissolved, then simmer for 1–2 minutes. Brush fish liberally with orange mixture and grill for 3–4 minutes each side, brushing with orange baste from time to time. Simmer remaining orange baste until it reduces and slightly thickens. Serve trout with orange sauce spooned over, baby new potatoes, minted peas and baby corn.
Serves 4

Per serve: 1114kJ/265Cals/5g fat

# Chicken with white wine and rosemary

I use a whole chicken which I then joint, but you can use chicken breasts, thighs, drumsticks or Marylands pieces as you wish. I like to use chicken on the bone as it gives a better flavour.

1 no.16 chicken, jointed, all skin and fat removed
1 large onion, chopped
1 clove garlic, crushed
1 large carrot, chopped
2 stalks celery, chopped
fresh rosemary sprigs, or 1 teaspoon dried rosemary
salt and pepper to taste
$1\frac{1}{2}$ cups white wine
1 cup chicken stock
1 tablespoon cornflour
1 teaspoon Parisian essence

Place chicken joints in one layer in a heavy-based saucepan or heatproof casserole. Sprinkle over vegetables and tuck the rosemary sprigs in among the joints. Season to taste with salt and pepper. Pour over white wine, cover and allow to marinate for 1 hour.

Pour over enough chicken stock to just cover the chicken pieces. Slowly bring to a gentle simmer, skimming off any scum that rises to the top. Cover and simmer until chicken is very tender, about 1 hour.

Remove chicken and vegetables from the pan with a slotted spoon and keep warm. Strain pan juices into a saucepan. Mix cornflour with a little water to a smooth paste. Mix in some of the hot pan juices until smooth. Add cornflour mixture to pan and enough Parisian essence to give a pleasing gravy-brown colour. Bring to the boil, stirring constantly until sauce thickens. Return chicken and vegetables to the pan, reduce heat and warm through. Serve immediately with potato and celery mash, broccoli and yellow squash.
Serves 6

Per serve: 919kJ/218Cals/6g fat

# Thai-style quail

4–8 quail (depending on size)
1½ tablespoons fish sauce
1½ tablespoons chopped fresh coriander
1 large clove garlic, sliced
1 tablespoon lemon juice
1/2 teaspoon grated fresh ginger
1/4 teaspoon chopped fresh chilli (or to taste)

Place the quail in a large dish. Combine remaining ingredients and pour over quail, making sure they are well covered in the marinade. Cover and refrigerate overnight.

Remove quail from refrigerator and allow to come to room temperature before cooking. Preheat oven to 200°C. Place quail in a non-stick roasting pan, resting on their sides. Roast for about 8 minutes, then remove from the oven, turn quail on their other sides, baste with marinade, return to the oven and continue cooking for a further 8 minutes or until the juices run clear when a skewer is inserted into the thickest part of their thigh. Serve with steamed rice, sweet chilli sauce and a salad.

Serves 4

Per serve: 842kJ/200Cals/7g fat

# Spatchcock with apple and apricot seasoning

4 spring onions, chopped
1/2 cup apple puree
60g dried apricots, chopped
15g roasted hazelnuts, chopped
2 tablespoons apple brandy
2 cups fresh wholemeal breadcrumbs
2 tablespoons chopped fresh mint
4 spatchcocks, skin removed
2 tablespoons soy sauce (salt-reduced)
1/4 cup redcurrant jelly

Preheat oven to 180°C. Place the spring onions, apple puree, apricots, hazelnuts, 1 tablespoon apple brandy, breadcrumbs and mint in a large bowl and combine well.

Wash spatchcocks inside and out. Pat dry with paper towel. Stuff birds with apple apricot seasoning and tie securely with kitchen string. Place in a large roasting pan. Place the soy sauce, redcurrant jelly and remaining apple brandy in a small saucepan and heat until combined. Brush over spatchcocks and cook for 20–30 minutes or until juices run clear when a skewer is inserted into the thickest part of the thigh. Serve either with crusty bread and salad or vegetables of choice.

*Note:* You can make a sauce from the pan juices by skimming any fat from the top and deglazing the pan with a little white wine or chicken stock. Strain this into the saucepan of redcurrant baste and simmer until it reduces and thickens slightly.
Serves 4

Per serve: 1585kJ/377Cals/11.9g fat

# Fillet steak with cherry sauce

4 slices fillet steak (about 180g each)
1 tablespoon red wine
2 tablespoons grain mustard
2 tablespoons blackberry jelly
2 tablespoons brandy
1 cup canned pitted morello cherries, drained, and 1/4 cup
   reserved syrup
salt and pepper to taste

Place the steak in a shallow dish. Combine the wine, mustard and jelly in a small pan and heat gently, stirring, until combined. Cool. Pour over steak. Cover and marinate for 1 hour.

    Drain steak and grill, or cook in a ridged frypan, until cooked to taste. Remove and keep warm. Strain remaining marinade and place in a small saucepan with the brandy and cherry syrup. Simmer until reduced by half. Add cherries and simmer until they are warmed through. Season to taste with salt and pepper. Serve steaks with cherries and sauce spooned over with baby new potatoes, carrots and broccoli.
Serves 4

Per serve: 1131kJ/269Cals/7g fat

# Peppered fillet of beef

750g fillet of beef
2 teaspoons red wine vinegar
1 tablespoon clear honey
1 tablespoon brandy
1 teaspoon soy sauce (salt-reduced)
1 teaspoon Worcestershire sauce
4 tablespoons cracked black pepper

Place the beef in a baking dish. Combine the vinegar, honey, brandy, soy sauce and Worcestershire sauce. Pour over beef, cover and marinade overnight.

Preheat oven to 200°C. Drain beef. Sprinkle pepper over a large flat plate and roll beef in it so that it is well covered. Place beef on a roasting rack in a pan to which 1 cup of water has been added. Roast 30–45 minutes or until cooked to taste. Serve with sugar snap peas, baked parsnips and boiled potatoes.
Serves 6

Per serve: 907kJ/216Cals/8.5g fat

# Steak with port and redcurrant sauce

1/4 cup port
2 tablespoons redcurrant jelly
1/2 stick cinnamon
zest 1 lemon
4 fillet steaks

Place the port, redcurrant jelly, cinnamon and lemon zest in a small saucepan and simmer gently for 5 minutes, or until reduced slightly. Grill steaks, or cook in a ridged non-stick frypan, until cooked to taste. Serve steaks with port sauce spooned over with vegetables of choice.
Serves 4

Per serve: 873kJ/208Cals/7g fat

# Roast rack of lamb with herb-mustard crust

2 racks lamb with 4 chops each
2 cloves garlic, crushed
2 tablespoons grain mustard
1/4 cup fresh wholemeal breadcrumbs
1 tablespoon lemon juice
1 teaspoon finely chopped rosemary
salt and pepper to taste

Preheat oven to 200°C. Trim lamb of any fat and skin. Combine remaining ingredients and spread over the backs of the racks. Place in a roasting tin and cook until done to taste—30–35 minutes for rare, 35–40 minutes for medium and 40–45 minutes for well done. Allow to stand covered in foil for 10 minutes before serving with minted new potatoes, peas and corn.
Serves 4

Per serve: 637kJ/151Cals/6g fat

# Stir-fried lamb with ginger and coriander

700g lamb fillets, cut into bite-sized pieces
3cm piece fresh ginger, peeled and sliced
2 cloves garlic, crushed
2 spring onions, chopped
1/4 cup dry sherry
1 tablespoon lemon juice
1/2 tablespoon soy sauce (salt-reduced)
1 teaspoon chopped fresh coriander

Combine all ingredients. Cover and marinate for at least 1 hour. Remove meat with a slotted spoon and reserve marinade.

Heat a non-stick wok or frypan over medium high heat. Stir-fry meat quickly until it changes colour. Remove meat from pan with a slotted spoon, leaving any juices in the pan. Add the marinade and simmer to reduce by half. Return meat to pan and heat through. Serve with boiled wild and brown rice blend and steamed vegetables. Serves 4

Per serve: 825kJ/196Cals/5.5g fat

# Lamb with herb-mustard crust

1 Trim Easy Carve lamb leg
1/4 cup grain mustard
1 large clove garlic, crushed
1 teaspoon chopped fresh thyme
1 teaspoon chopped fresh marjoram
1/2 cup fine breadcrumbs

Preheat oven to 180°C. Weigh lamb to calculate cooking time and trim off any remaining fat. Combine the mustard, garlic and herbs and smear all over the lamb. Sprinkle the breadcrumbs on a large flat plate and roll lamb in them to coat well.

Place the lamb on a rack in a roasting pan to which 1 cup of water has been added. Roast for 20–25 minutes per 500g for rare, 25–30 minutes per 500g for medium and 30–35 minutes per 500g for well done. Allow to stand covered with foil for 10–15 minutes before carving. Serve with potatoes, parsnips and pumpkin braised in the oven in a covered dish with a little white wine, garlic and freshly chopped herbs—place vegetables in oven 40 minutes before the end of cooking time.
Serves 6

Per serve: 858kJ/204Cals/5.8g fat

# Cajun pork with fresh peach salsa

You can buy premixed cajun spices in jars from the herb and spice sections of major supermarkets. I find them quick and convenient to use.

2 whole pork fillets (about 750g), trimmed of any fat
2 tablespoons prepared cajun spices
4 ripe peaches
2 tablespoons orange juice
1 teaspoon brown sugar
1 teaspoon chopped chilli
1 tablespoon finely chopped coriander

Place pork in a glass dish. Sprinkle over cajun spices and rub in, making sure the meat is well coated. Cover and refrigerate for 2 hours.

Preheat oven to 190°C. Place pork on a roasting rack, tucking the thin tails under so the fillets are an even thickness for all their lengths. Place rack in a roasting pan and add 1 cup of water. Roast for 20 minutes. Baste with pan juices and continue roasting for a further 20 minutes or until pork is cooked. Allow to stand for 10 minutes.

While the pork is cooking prepare the peach salsa. Place peaches in a bowl and pour over boiling water. Stand for 1 minute, then drain. Peel off peach skins, halve, remove stones and finely chop flesh. Combine with remaining ingredients. Slice pork and serve with peach salsa and a green salad.

Serves 4

Per serve: 1030kJ/245Cals/1.9g fat

# Butterfly pork with apricots and prunes

4 New Fashioned butterfly steaks, trimmed of fat
salt and pepper to taste
60g dried apricots
60g dried pitted prunes
1 onion, sliced
8 small new potatoes
1/4 teaspoon cinnamon
1/8 teaspoon ground cloves
1/2 cup chicken stock

Season the pork steaks with salt and pepper and brown in a non-stick frypan. Transfer to a casserole dish. Arrange apricots, prunes, onion and new potatoes over pork. Combine the cinnamon, cloves and stock and pour over meat. Cover and bake for 30–40 minutes or until pork is tender. Serve with a green vegetable.
Serves 4

Per serve: 1327kJ/316Cals/3g fat

# Veal roast with apricot glaze

1kg nut of veal
2 tablespoons apricot conserve
2 tablespoons soy sauce (salt-reduced)
1 tablespoon apricot brandy
1 tablespoon honey
1 tablespoon white wine vinegar
1 tablespoon lemon juice
1/8 teaspoon cardamom
1/8 teaspoon cinnamon
salt and pepper to taste

Preheat oven to 180°C. Place the veal on a rack in a roasting pan to which 1 cup water has been added. Combine remaining ingredients in a small saucepan and bring to the boil, stirring constantly. Remove from the heat and brush over roast, coating it well. Roast for 1¼ hours or until veal is tender and cooked through, basting with glaze every 15 minutes. Allow to stand covered with foil for 10–15 minutes before carving. Serve with baby new potatoes, spinach and mushrooms.
Serves 6

Per serve: 824kJ/196Cals/2g fat

# Veal fillet with blackberry-herb crust

750g veal loin roast, trimmed of any fat
salt and cracked black pepper to taste
1/3 cup brown sugar
2 tablespoons blackberry conserve
1/4 cup chopped mixed herbs such as parsley, sorrel, sage and rosemary
1/4 cup concentrated veal or vegetable stock

Place the veal in a baking dish. Season with salt and pepper. Combine the sugar, conserve and herbs and spread over veal. Cover and marinate for several hours. Preheat oven to 180°C. Place veal on a rack in a roasting pan to which 1 cup of water has been added. Roast veal for 45–60 minutes or until cooked through, basting with stock every 15 minutes. Allow to stand, covered in foil, for 10–15 minutes before carving. Serve with yellow button squash and asparagus.
Serves 4

Per serve: 831kJ/198Cals/1g fat

# Mushroom, asparagus and artichoke lasagna

1 large onion, chopped
1 large clove garlic, crushed
1/2 cup chopped parsley
1/3 cup vegetable stock or dry white wine
250g flat mushrooms, chopped
$2\frac{1}{2}$ tablespoons cornflour
$2\frac{1}{2}$ cups skim milk
salt and pepper to taste
1 bunch asparagus spears
6 instant lasagna sheets
200g jar artichoke hearts, drained
14 cup freshly grated Parmesan cheese

Preheat oven to 180°C. Saute the onion, garlic and parsley in the stock or wine in a large heavy-based saucepan over medium heat, until softened. Add the mushrooms and continue to cook until mushrooms soften. Remove from the heat.

Blend the cornflour with a little of the milk to form a smooth milky mix. Add remaining milk to the mushroom mixture and stir over medium heat until milk is just below simmering point. Stir in the cornflour mixture and cook, stirring continuously, until the sauce boils and thickens. Remove from the heat and season to taste with salt and pepper.

Steam or microwave the asparagus until cooked but still crisp. Place a layer of mushroom sauce in the bottom of an ovenproof serving dish. Cover with a layer of lasagna, then a layer of asparagus spears and artichokes, then cover this with mushroom sauce and then lasagna. Continue layering, finishing with a layer of mushroom sauce. Sprinkle with Parmesan cheese and bake in the oven for 25–30 minutes or until piping hot and lasagna is tender. Serve with a mixed green salad and crusty bread.
Serves 6

Per serve: 579kJ/138Cals/1.7g fat

# Ricotta, spinach and pine nut stuffed pancakes

1/2 cup plain flour
pinch salt (optional)
1 large egg
1 egg white
300ml (1¼ cups) skim milk (approx.)
250g frozen chopped spinach, thawed and drained
250g low-fat ricotta cheese
1 tablespoon lemon juice
2 tablespoons pine nuts, toasted
salt and pepper to taste

Sift the flour and salt into a large bowl. Beat the egg and egg white together until combined. Stir in the milk. Add to flour a little at a time, stirring to achieve a pouring batter (you may have to add a little more milk to achieve this). Heat the spinach in a small pan or microwave until hot, drain thoroughly and mix with the ricotta, lemon juice and pine nuts. Season to taste with salt and pepper. Place, covered, into a low oven to warm through.

Heat a small, non-stick frying pan over medium heat. Pour in 1/4 cup of batter. Swirl batter around the pan to cover the bottom. As soon as the base is set flip it over to cook the other side. Remove from pan and keep warm. Repeat with remaining mixture.

Place spoonfuls of ricotta mixture onto pancakes, roll up and serve with a green salad, and sliced tomatoes sprinkled with balsamic vinegar and chopped fresh basil.
Serves 6

Per serve: 657kJ/154Cals/6.8g fat

# Spicy marinated tofu and vegetable stir-fry

375g firm tofu, diced
1/3 cup soy sauce (salt-reduced)
1/4 cup honey
1/4 cup Worcestershire sauce
2 tablespoons tomato sauce
1/4 teaspoon minced fresh ginger
1/4 teaspoon minced fresh chilli
1 onion, cut into petals
1 clove garlic, crushed
1 small carrot, sliced diagonally
1 stalk celery, sliced diagonally
4 yellow button squash, sliced
1 small red capsicum, cored, seeded and chopped
1/4 cup vegetable stock or dry white wine

Place the diced tofu into a bowl. Combine the soy sauce, honey, sauces, ginger and chilli. Mix well. Pour over the tofu and stir to ensure that it is well coated. Cover and refrigerate for 2 hours.

Stir-fry the vegetables in the stock until they are just cooked. Add the tofu and marinade to the pan and toss until heated through. Serve with steamed rice and some chopped cashew nuts sprinkled on top if liked.
Serves 6

Per serve: 631kJ/150Cals/3.29g fat

# Wild rice, vegetable and cashew nut salad

4 cups cooked long grain and wild rice blend
1/3 cup diced yellow capsicum
1/3 cup diced red capsicum
1/3 cup diced green capsicum
1/3 cup sweet corn kernels
1/2 cup chopped celery
1 small red onion, finely chopped
1 cup chopped parsley
1/4 cup fish sauce
1 tablespoon lemon juice
1 tablespoon sweet chilli sauce
1/2 tablespoon soy sauce
1/2 tablespoon brown sugar
1 teaspoon chopped fresh basil (optional)
2 tablespoons chopped fresh parsley for garnish
30g cashew nuts, chopped

Mix the rice and vegetables together well in a large bowl. Combine remaining ingredients except the extra parsley and nuts. Pour over rice mixture and toss through. Serve sprinkled with parsley and cashew nuts.
Serves 6

Per serve: 922kJ/219Cals/3.8g fat

# Index

Aerobics 39
Almond, date and rice pudding 211
Apple and blackberry crumble 224
Apple and mustard dressing 192
Apple and onion sauce 199
Apple and walnut scone loaf 236
Apple snow 218
Apricot pork kebabs 108
Apricot yoghurt smoothie 68
Artichokes with spicy yoghurt dip 170
Asparagus mornay 80
Atherosclerosis 5

Baked pork fillet with tomato
  sherry glaze 109
Baking 228–38
  Apple and walnut scone loaf 236
  Banana honey drop scones 233
  Banana pecan fudge squares 231
  Date, walnut and banana bread
    237
  Lancashire parkin 229
  Low-fat walnut brownies 228
  Mixed fruit tea bread 238
  Pumpkin bread 232
  Quick beer damper 230
  Quick corn bread 234
  Simple date and pecan loaf 235
Balsamic cherry pickle 197
Banana and cheese pita pockets 79
Banana honey drop scones 233
Banana pecan fudge squares 231
Barbecued chicken with lemon and
  paprika 118
Barbecued tipsy chicken 118

Barbecuing 59
Beans with rice and vegetables 152
Beef 91–7
  Beef and capsicum salad 81
  Beef partners 97
  Beef stock 91
  Beef, vegetables and noodles 92
  Beef with snow peas and rice 156
  Capsicum stuffed with beef and
    mushrooms 157
  Fillet steak with cherry sauce
    249
  Guilt-free spaghetti bolognese
    162
  Marinated rump steak 96
  Meatballs with tomato sauce 95
  Old-fashioned shepherd's pie 93
  Peppered fillet of beef 250
  Steak with port and redcurrant
    sauce 251
  Stir-fried beef and vegetables 94
  Thai beef salad 97
Black beans, capsicum and
  coriander 178
Body fat 3–9, 10, 12, 13, 16, 21,
  23, 24, 38, 41–7, 48
Body mass index 6, 7–8
Bouillabaisse 244
Braised ocean salmon 243
Breakfasts 68–76
  Apricot yoghurt smoothie 68
  Cheese and bean muffins 74
  Chicken sausages and baked
    beans 76

Corn, ham and mushroom bagels 74
Easy breakfast kedgeree 75
Fruit muesli 70
Mango yoghurt breakfast drink 69
Mixed berry smoothie 68
Mixed fruit breakfast cocktail 69
Pancakes with mushrooms, ham and corn 73
Pancakes with yoghurt and berries 72
Rice with apple and yoghurt 71
Butterfly pork with apricots and prunes 255

Cajun chicken 117
Cajun pork with fresh peach salsa 254
Calcium 26–7
Capsicum stuffed with beef and mushrooms 157
Caramel grapes with vanilla yoghurt 220
Caramel oranges 220
Casseroling 60–1
Cheese and bean muffins 74
Cheese and herb morsels 209
Cheesy capsicum spread 206
Chicken and mushroom risotto 159
Chicken in a pot 115
Chicken meatballs with pasta 165
Chicken noodle salad 84
Chicken poached in orange sauce 122
Chicken sausages and baked beans 76
Chicken stock 114
Chicken tikka 121
Chicken with curry mango glaze 127

Chicken with mustard and tarragon 122
Chicken with plum-soy glaze 128
Chicken with teriyaki glaze 123
Chicken with walnuts and apricot sauce 125
Chicken with walnut crust 126
Chicken with white wine and rosemary 246
Chickpea and vegetable curry 181
Chickpea snack 203
Chilli coriander snapper 140
Chilli orange dipping sauce 193
Cholesterol 5, 28, 30
Cider pork kebabs 106
Coleslaw dressing 197
Corn, ham and mushroom bagels 74
Corn, potato and broccoli soup 78
Coronary artery disease 4–5
Cottage cheese, pineapple and gherkin dip 204
Crab cakes with cucumber relish 87
Crab, cheese and cucumber cups 210
Cracked wheat and tomato salad 186
Creamy horseradish dressing 189
Creamy salad dressing 188
Crunchy baked apples 212
Crunchy pear cobbler 227
Curried yoghurt dressing 188

Date, walnut and banana bread 237
Deep sea perch poached in tequila 139
Desserts 211–27
Almond, date and rice pudding 211

Apple and blackberry crumble 224

Apple snow 218

Caramel grapes with vanilla yoghurt 220

Caramel oranges 220

Crunchy baked apples 212

Crunchy pear cobbler 227

Figs poached in red wine 216

Fruit salad with sherried yoghurt 224

Fruit-topped pavlova 225

Low-fat butterscotch sauce 213

Pear and cinnamon parcels 226

Pears and ginger self-saucing pudding 217

Ricotta with raspberry coulis 221

Spiced fruit compote 215

Strawberries with meringue topping 219

Strawberry delight 223

Sultana, ginger and ricotta pastries 214

Summer pudding 222

Vanilla custard 227

Vanilla topping 212

Diabetes, mature onset 5

Dietary fibre 23

Diets 17

Easy breakfast kedgeree 75

Eggs 71

Entertaining 239–61

  Bouillabaisse 244

  Braised ocean salmon 243

  Butterfly pork with apricots and prunes 255

  Cajun pork with fresh peach salsa 254

  Chicken with white wine and rosemary 246

  Fillet steak with cherry sauce 249

  Grilled Atlantic salmon with fennel and walnuts 242

  Lamb with herb mustard crust 253

  Mushroom, asparagus and artichoke lasagna 258

  Peppered fillet of beef 250

  Polynesian salmon and tomato salad 240

  Rainbow trout with orange and ginger 245

  Ricotta, spinach and pine nut stuffed pancakes 259

  Roast rack of lamb with herb-mustard crust 251

  Salmon ramekins with soy ginger dressing 239

  Seafood pasta 241

  Spatchcocks with apple and apricot seasoning 248

  Spicy marinated tofu and vegetable stir-fry 260

  Steak with port and redcurrant sauce 251

  Stir-fried lamb with ginger and coriander 252

  Thai-style quail 247

  Veal fillet with blackberry-herb crust 257

  Veal roast with apricot glaze 256

  Wild rice, vegetable and cashew nut salad 261

Exercise 38–40

Exercise combinations 40

Fat 10–15, 16–22, 23, 24, 25, 28, 29, 38–40, 41, 45, 46, 48, 49,

50, 51, 52, 53, 54, 56, 57, 59, 63, 67
Fat-burning exercise 39–40
Fat cells 6, 13, 16, 17, 18
Fat guide 29, 30
Fat loss eating plan 48–58
Fat quiz 11
Fatty acids
  Essential 4,
  Omega–3 30
  Omega–6 30
  Saturated 19, 29
  Unsaturated 25, 28, 29
Figs poached in red wine 216
Fillet steak with cherry sauce 249
Fish stock 130
Fish with mango and mint 149
Five food groups 56–57
Food labels 47
Fruit muesli 70
Fruit salad with sherried yoghurt 224
Fruit-topped pavlova 225

Garlic pita crisps 204
Grilled Atlantic salmon with fennel and walnuts 242
Grilled octopus 147
Grilled tuna with potato and celery mash 138
Grilled veal steaks with wine-rosemary baste 111
Grilling 60
Guilt-free potato chips 202
Guilt-free spaghetti bolognese 162

Ham and orange slaw 83
Ham, mushroom and zucchini pasta 160
Hardening of the arteries 5

Heart disease 4–5
Hearty pumpkin soup 177
Hearty vegetable soup 175
High blood pressure see hypertension
Honey ginger salad dressing 193
Honey prawns 133
Hypertension 5, 30

Iced lettuce and cucumber soup 176
Iron 27
Italian chicken 117
Italian-style veal casserole 110

Jacket potatoes with beans and ham 89
Jogging 39

Kidney disease 5

Lamb 98–103
  Lamb and vegetable stew 100
  Lamb partners 102
  Lamb pilaf 99
  Lamb stuffed with apricot and coriander 103
  Lamb with herb-mustard crust 253
  Lebanese-style lamb meatballs 101
  Mini roast with orange sauce 98
  Roast rack of lamb with herb-mustard crust 251
  Spicy lamb leg steaks 102
  Stir-fried lamb with ginger and coriander 252
Lancashire parkin 229
Lebanese-style lamb meatballs 101
Lemon Dijon dressing 189

Lemon grass chicken 120
Ling and vegetable casserole 136
Ling in lettuce parcels 131
Lipogenic enzymes 16, 17
Lipolytic enzymes 16, 17, 38, 40
Low-fat butterscotch sauce 213
Low-fat walnut brownies 228
Lunch dishes 77–90
  Asparagus mornay 80
  Banana, cheese and pita pockets 79
  Beef and capsicum salad 81
  Chicken noodle salad 84
  Corn, potato and broccoli soup 78
  Crab cakes with cucumber relish 87
  Ham and orange slaw 83
  Jacket potatoes with beans and ham 89
  Potato with chicken and corn 88
  Prawns and crab salad 82
  Pumpkin and apple soup 77
  Quick fish lunch 90
  Salmon burgers 86
  Tuna, corn and lettuce pockets 80
  Warm baby octopus salad 85

Magnesium 28
Manganese 28
Mango salsa 195
Mango yoghurt breakfast drink 69
Marinated rump steak 96
Marinated tofu and vegetables 179
Marinades, rubs and glazes:
  Dry rub marinades for chicken 125
  Dry rub for barbecued steak 96
  Garlic lemon marinade for chicken 126
  Glaze for lamb or pork 107
  Marinades for chicken 121
  Marinade for oily fish 138
  Rub for veal 113
  Thai flavoured pork marinade 105
Mature onset diabetes 5
Meat 59, 60, 61, 62
Meatballs with tomato sauce 95
Mediterranean fish casserole 146
Menopause 7
Metabolism 7, 10, 16, 17, 25, 26, 28, 40, 41, 42, 50, 54
Microwaved jacket potatoes 176
Microwaved pappadums 182
Microwaving 60–1
Millet, bean and capsicum pilaf 187
Mini roast with orange sauce 98
Mixed berry smoothie 68
Mixed fruit breakfast cocktail 69
Mixed fruit tea bread 238
Mixed vegetable parcels 180
Mixed vegetable pasta bake 172
Mornay sauce 200
Mushroom, asparagus and artichoke lasagna 258
Mushroom pâté 205
Mussels with tomato and garlic 143

Nutrition 23–37, 47, 57

Obesity 6, 7
Old-fashioned shepherd's pie 93
Osteoarthritis 6

Pancakes with mushrooms, ham and corn 73

Pancakes with yoghurt and berries 72

Pasta and rice 151–69
    Beans with rice and vegetables 152
    Beef, vegetables and noodles 92
    Beef with snow peas and rice 156
    Capsicum stuffed with beef and mushrooms 157
    Chicken and mushroom risotto 159
    Chicken meatballs with pasta 165
    Chicken noodle salad 84
    Guilt-free spaghetti bolognese 162
    Ham, mushroom and zucchini pasta 160
    Pasta with artichokes, sun-dried tomatoes and chilli 169
    Pasta with chicken livers 161
    Pasta with ham and avocado 167
    Pasta with mushrooms and beans 173
    Pasta with spinach and pine nut sauce 168
    Quick tuna and tomato pasta 151
    Rice with chickpeas and corn 158
    Rice with crab and corn 154
    Savoury rice with vegetables 153
    Seafood pasta 241
    Seafood rice salad 155
    Tomato, anchovy and olive pasta 166
    Tuna, mushroom and artichoke pasta 164
    Zucchini, capsicum and sour cream pasta 163

Pear and cinnamon parcels 226
Pearl perch with honey mustard glaze 145
Pears and ginger self-saucing pudding 217
Peppered fillet of beef 250
Piquant prawns 142
Piquant sauce 191
Pizza-flavoured popcorn 202
Polynesian salmon and tomato salad 240
Pork 104–9
    Apricot pork kebabs 108
    Baked pork fillet with tomato sherry glaze 109
    Butterfly pork with apricots and prunes 255
    Cajun pork with fresh peach salsa 254
    Cider pork kebabs 106
    Ham and orange slaw 83
    Ham, mushroom and zucchini pasta 160
    Pasta with ham and avocado 167
    Pork chops with redcurrant glaze 107
    Pork partners 106
    Soy sherry pork steaks 105
    Spicy roast pork 104
    Thai flavoured pork marinade 105
Port and redcurrant sauce 198
Potato with chicken and corn 88
Potatoes with chilli beans 182
Poultry 61, 62, 114–29
    Barbecued chicken with lemon and paprika 118
    Barbecued tipsy chicken 118
    Cajun chicken 117

Chicken and mushroom risotto 159
Chicken in a pot 115
Chicken meatballs with pasta 165
Chicken noodle salad 84
Chicken poached in orange sauce 122
Chicken sausages and baked beans 76
Chicken stock 114
Chicken tikka 121
Chicken with curry mango glaze 127
Chicken with mustard and tarragon 122
Chicken with plum-soy glaze 128
Chicken with teriyaki glaze 123
Chicken with walnuts and apricot sauce 125
Chicken with walnut crust 126
Chicken with white wine and rosemary 246
Dry-rub marinades for chicken 125
Garlic lemon marinade for chicken 126
Italian chicken 117
Lemon grass chicken 120
Marinades for chicken 121
Pasta with chicken livers 161
Potato with chicken and corn 88
Poultry partners 116
Spatchcocks with apple and apricot seasoning 248
Spatchcocks with garlic and coriander 128
Spicy chicken parcels 116
Steamed tarragon chicken with vegetables 129

Tandoori chicken 124
Thai chicken salad 119
Thai-style quail 247
Pumpkin and apple soup 77
Pumpkin bread 232

Quick beer damper 230
Quick corn bread 234
Quick fish lunch 90
Quick tuna and tomato pasta 151

Rainbow trout with orange and ginger 245
Redcurrant-mint sauce 199
Retinopathy 5
Rice with apple and yoghurt 71
Rice with crab and corn 154
Rice with chickpeas and corn 158
Ricotta, spinach and pine nut stuffed pancakes 259
Ricotta with raspberry coulis 221
Roast rack of lamb with herb-mustard crust 251
Roasted yellow capsicum sauce 195
Roasting/baking 61–2

Salad dressings, sauces, salsas and chutneys 188–200
Apple and mustard dressing 192
Apple and onion sauce 199
Balsamic cherry pickle 197
Chilli orange dipping sauce 193
Coleslaw dressing 194
Creamy horseradish dressing 189
Creamy salad dressing 188
Curried yoghurt dressing 188
For barbecued fish 145
For grilled lamb 100
Honey ginger salad dressing 193

Lemon Dijon dressing 189
Mango salsa 195
Mornay sauce 200
Piquant sauce 191
Port and redcurrant sauce 198
Redcurrant-mint sauce 199
Roasted yellow capsicum sauce 195
Sesame soy garlic dressing 190
Spiced tomato jam 196
Spicy tomato dressing 190
Sweet chilli sauce 198
Tomato sauce  192
Vegetarian bolognese sauce 184
Wild rice, vegetable and cashew
    nut salad 261
Yoghurt dill dressing 191
Salads
    Beef and capsicum salad 81
    Chicken noodle salad 84
    Ham and orange slaw 83
    Prawns and crab salad 82
    Seafood rice salad 155
    Thai beef salad 97
    Thai chicken salad 119
    Warm baby octopus salad 85
Salmon and cucumber bites 206
Salmon burgers 86
Salmon dip 201
Salmon ramekins with soy ginger
    dressing 239
Salmon steaks with cucumber and
    dill 144
Savoury rice with vegetables 153
Seafood 59, 60, 61, 62, 130–50
    Baste for baked, barbecued or
        grilled fish 148
    Bouillabaisse 244
    Braised ocean salmon 243
    Chilli coriander snapper 140

Crab cakes with cucumber relish
    87
Deep sea perch poached in
    tequila 139
Fish stock 130
Fish with mango and mint 149
Grilled Atlantic salmon with
    fennel and walnuts 242
Grilled octopus 147
Grilled tuna with potato and
    celery mash 138
Honey prawns 133
Ling and vegetable casserole 136
Ling in lettuce parcels 131
Mediterranean fish casserole 146
Mussels with tomato and garlic
    143
Pearl perch with honey mustard
    glaze 145
Piquant prawns 142
Polynesian salmon and tomato
    salad 240
Prawn and crab salad 82
Quick fish lunch 90
Rainbow trout with orange and
    ginger 245
Salmon and cucumber bites 206
Salmon burgers 86
Salmon dip 201
Salmon ramekins with soy
    ginger dressing 239
Salmon steaks with cucumber
    and dill 144
Seafood pasta 241
Seafood rice salad 155
Seafood stir-fry 150
Spicy Indian seafood 134
Snapper and vegetable bake 137
Snapper and vegetable casserole
    149

Sweet and sour fish parcels 135
Swordfish kebabs 141
Tuna, corn and lettuce pockets 80
Tuna, mushroom and artichoke pasta 164
Warm baby octopus salad 85
Whiting with lemon and dill baste 148
Sesame soy garlic dressing 190
Simple date and pecan loaf 235
Snacks 201–10
  Cheese and herb morsels 209
  Cheesy capsicum spread 206
  Chickpea snack 203
  Cottage cheese, pineapple and gherkin dip 204
  Crab, cheese and cucumber cups 210
  Garlic pita crisps 204
  Guilt-free potato chips 202
  Mushroom pâté 205
  Pizza-flavoured popcorn 202
  Salmon and cucumber bites 206
  Salmon dip 201
  Snow peas stuffed with cheese and prawns 207
  Spicy crab dip 203
  Spicy eggplant garlic dip 201
  Spicy tomato dip 210
  Sun-dried tomato and basil dip 208
  Sweet potato and pumpkin crisps 209
  Three bean dip 207
Snapper and vegetable bake 137
Snapper and vegetable casserole 149
Snow peas stuffed with cheese and prawns 207

Soups
  Corn, potato and broccoli soup 78
  Hearty pumpkin soup 177
  Hearty vegetable soup 175
  Iced lettuce and cucumber soup 176
  Pumpkin and apple soup 77
Soy sherry pork steaks 105
Spatchcocks with apple and apricot seasoning 248
Spatchcocks with garlic and coriander 128
Spiced fruit compote 215
Spiced tomato jam 196
Spicy chicken parcels 116
Spicy chickpeas and potatoes 181
Spicy crab dip 203
Spicy eggplant garlic dip 201
Spicy Indian seafood 134
Spicy lamb leg steaks 102
Spicy marinated tofu and vegetable stir-fry 260
Spicy roast pork 104
Spicy tomato dip 210
Spicy tomato dressing 190
Spicy tomato jam 196
Steak with port and redcurrant sauce 251
Steamed tarragon chicken with vegetables 129
Steaming 62
Stir-fried beef and vegetables 94
Stir-fried lamb with ginger and coriander 252
Stir-frying 62
Strawberries with meringue topping 219
Strawberry delight 223
Stroke 5

Sultana, ginger and ricotta pastries 214

Summer pudding 222

Sun-dried tomato and basil dip 208

Sweet and sour fish parcels 135

Sweet chilli sauce 198

Sweet potato and pumpkin crisps 209

Swordfish kebabs 141

Tandoori chicken 124

Thai beef salad 97

Thai chicken salad 119

Thai-style quail 247

Three bean dip 207

Tomato, anchovy and olive pasta 166

Tomato and artichoke pasta sauce 174

Tomato, bean and mushroom casserole 171

Tomato, corn and pea curry 185

Tomato sauce 192

Tuna, corn and lettuce pockets 80

Tuna, mushroom and artichoke pasta 164

Unsaturated fatty acids 28–29

Vanilla custard 227

Vanilla topping 212

Veal 110–13

Grilled veal steaks with wine-rosemary baste 111

Italian-style veal casserole 110

Veal and artichoke casserole 112

Veal fillet with blackberry-herb crust 257

Veal marsala 113

Veal partners 111

Veal roast with apricot glaze 256

Vegetable dishes 170–87

Artichokes with spicy yoghurt dip 170

Asparagus mornay 80

Black beans, capsicum and coriander 178

Chickpea and vegetable curry 181

Cracked wheat and tomato salad 186

Hearty pumpkin soup 177

Hearty vegetable soup 175

Iced lettuce and cucumber soup 176

Marinated tofu and vegetables 179

Microwaved jacket potatoes 176

Millet, bean and capsicum pilaf 187

Mixed vegetable parcels 180

Mixed vegetable pasta bake 172

Mushroom, asparagus and artichoke lasagna 258

Pasta with artichokes, sun-dried tomatoes and chilli 169

Pasta with mushrooms and beans 173

Pasta with spinach and pine nut sauce 168

Potatoes with chilli beans 182

Rice with chickpeas and corn 158

Ricotta, spinach and pine nut stuffed pancakes 259

Spicy chickpeas and potatoes 181

Spicy marinated tofu and vegetable stir-fry 260

Tomato and artichoke pasta sauce 174

Tomato, bean and mushroom casserole 171

Tomato, corn and pea curry 185
Vegetable stir-fry with almonds 183
Vegetarian bolognese sauce 184
Wild rice, vegetable and cashew
nut salad 261
Zucchini, capsicum and sour
cream pasta 163

Waist measurement risk 4
Walking 39

Warm baby octopus salad 85
Weight for height 8
Whiting with lemon and dill baste 148
Wild rice, vegetable and cashew
nut salad 261

Yoghurt dill dressing 191

Zucchini, capsicum and sour
cream pasta 163